Surendra Akash

Adverse drug reactions due to cancer chemotherapy

Adverse drug reactions due to cancer
chemotherapy in a tertiary care centre

LAP LAMBERT Academic Publishing

Impressum / Imprint

Bibliografische Information der Deutschen Nationalbibliothek: Die Deutsche Nationalbibliothek verzeichnet diese Publikation in der Deutschen Nationalbibliografie; detaillierte bibliografische Daten sind im Internet über http://dnb.d-nb.de abrufbar.

Alle in diesem Buch genannten Marken und Produktnamen unterliegen warenzeichen-, marken- oder patentrechtlichem Schutz bzw. sind Warenzeichen oder eingetragene Warenzeichen der jeweiligen Inhaber. Die Wiedergabe von Marken, Produktnamen, Gebrauchsnamen, Handelsnamen, Warenbezeichnungen u.s.w. in diesem Werk berechtigt auch ohne besondere Kennzeichnung nicht zu der Annahme, dass solche Namen im Sinne der Warenzeichen- und Markenschutzgesetzgebung als frei zu betrachten wären und daher von jedermann benutzt werden dürften.

Bibliographic information published by the Deutsche Nationalbibliothek: The Deutsche Nationalbibliothek lists this publication in the Deutsche Nationalbibliografie; detailed bibliographic data are available in the Internet at http://dnb.d-nb.de.

Any brand names and product names mentioned in this book are subject to trademark, brand or patent protection and are trademarks or registered trademarks of their respective holders. The use of brand names, product names, common names, trade names, product descriptions etc. even without a particular marking in this works is in no way to be construed to mean that such names may be regarded as unrestricted in respect of trademark and brand protection legislation and could thus be used by anyone.

Coverbild / Cover image: www.ingimage.com

Verlag / Publisher:
LAP LAMBERT Academic Publishing
ist ein Imprint der / is a trademark of
AV Akademikerverlag GmbH & Co. KG
Heinrich-Böcking-Str. 6-8, 66121 Saarbrücken, Deutschland / Germany
Email: info@lap-publishing.com

Herstellung: siehe letzte Seite /
Printed at: see last page
ISBN: 978-3-8433-9037-8

Zugl. / Approved by: Panaji, Goa University, 2011

Surendra Akash

Adverse drug reactions due to cancer chemotherapy

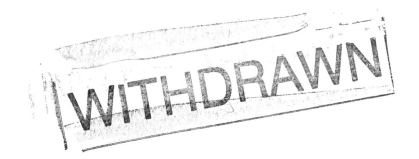

ADVERSE DRUG REACTIONS DUE TO CANCER CHEMOTHERAPY IN TERTIARY CARE CENTRE, GOA MEDICAL COLLEGE AND HOSPITAL BAMBOLIM GOA

Dr. Surendra S. Akash

M.B.B.S

M.D.(pharmacology)

Assistant Professor

Department of Pharmacology

**TRAVANCORE MEDICAL COLLEGE
KOLLAM
KERALA**

ADVERSE DRUG REACTIONS DUE TO CANCER CHEMOTHERAPY IN TERTIARY CARE CENTRE, GOA MEDICAL COLLEGE AND HOSPITAL BAMBOLIM GOA

DISSERTATION SUBMITTED IN THE PARTIAL

FULFILLMENT OF REQUIREMENTS OF THE

AWARD OF MD {PHARMACOLOGY}

BY

DR. SURENDRA. S. AKASH

Done under the guidance of

DR. SUSHAMA A. BHOUNSULE M.D.

Director Professor

Department of Pharmacology

GOA MEDICAL COLLEGE

GOA

Acknowledgements

It is with immense delight that I take this opportunity to express deep gratitude and indebtness to my esteemed guide and teacher Dr. Sushama. A. Bhounsule, Director Professor, Department of Pharmacology, Goa Medical College, Bambolim, Goa for her precious guidance and supervision provided during course of this study.

I am also grateful to Dr. J.S.C. Pereira, Director Professor and Head, Department of Pharmacology, Goa Medical College, Bambolim-Goa for his unvarying encouragement and support.

I am also indebted to Mr. M S. Kulkarni, Statistician, Department of Preventive and Social Medicine, Goa Medical College, Bambolim, Goa, for helping me in the keen observation of the cases.

I would be failing in my duty if I do not credit the efforts of paramedical staff, non-teaching staff and colleagues.

I owe a special thanks to Dr. V. N. Jindal, Dean, Goa Medical College and Hospital, Bambolim, Goa, for granting me to conduct this study in the institute.

I also appreciate the wholesome cooperation extended by the resident doctors and the nursing staff of the institute.

It is indeed a fudiciary obligation to acknowledge my gratitude to all my patients, who inspite of their continuing agony and distress have co-operated and participated in this study without which this study would have been just a chimera.

Above all, this work would not have been complete without the grace and blessings of God; to whom I offer my sincere prayers.

Dr. Surendra. S Akash
Assistant Professor
Dept. of Pharmacology
Travancore Medical College
Kollam
Kerala
Email-
drsurendraakash@yahoo.com

Index

INTRODUCTION

In the past 4 decades, the practice of cancer medicine has dramatically changed, as curative treatments have been identified for a number of previously fatal malignancies. New drugs have entered clinical use for cancer presentations that were previously either untreatable or amenable only to local therapies such as surgery and irradiations. At present, adjuvant chemotherapy routinely follows local treatment of breast, colorectal and lung cancer and chemotherapy is employed as a part of multinodal approach to the initial treatment of many other tumours. With this approach in mind, one has to be aware of the multiplicity of adverse effects which will be associated with the combination anticancer drugs in cancer patients correctly. In the speciality of oncology, when the chance of a cure from cancer is high, a medicine's toxicity becomes more acceptable to patients and clinicians. Successful treatment depends on the effective management and prevention of adverse drug reactions to the cytotoxic agents. Until now, the basis of drug safety monitoring has largely remained spontaneous adverse drug reaction (ADR) reporting. This method is, nevertheless, limited mainly by underreporting, which does not allow medical care assessment of ADRs' real impact. Most hospitals identify an ADR by spontaneous or stimulated reporting, leading to a systematically underestimated frequency of ADRs. Chart review identifies considerably more ADRs, but it is not sufficiently cost effective for routine use. Another approach is the computerized detection[1]. The principle is to look for signals suggesting the possible presence of an ADR from hospital information systems. The databases most often used are pharmacy and laboratory databases, but also medical administrative databases, with in particular data about diagnoses and therapeutic interventions. The querying of computerized databases is interesting for generating pharmacovigilance signals, but alone they do not permit estimation of the real frequency of adverse drug reactions (ADRs)[1]. In fact, no source of ADR identification (spontaneous reporting or computerized detection) is really exhaustive. Nevertheless, simultaneous use of these sources should improve detection of ADRs and thus provide better knowledge of the impact of hospital ADRs. Adverse drug reactions (ADRs) related to cancer drugs are an important cause of morbidity and mortality[2]. Serious or potentially fatal ADRs are often detected after cancer drugs are widely used in oncology practice. Premarketing clinical trials are

1

designed primarily to identify benefits and common side effects of new drugs; however, the size of these studies generally does not exceed 3,000 patients, limiting the likelihood of detecting rare ADRs before approval. Oncology drug–associated ADRs are particularly important to consider, given that these drugs may be especially likely to cause ADRs because they are designed to be cytotoxic and thus often injure normal cells in addition to the malignant cells[2]. When previously unidentified but serious ADRs are reported after the drug has been approved by the US Food and Drug Administration (FDA), information dissemination occurs through revised package inserts (PIs), so-called Dear Doctor letters, and/or publications in medical journals. Despite medical professionals' and patients' dependence on this information to ensure safe pharmaceutical usage, ADR reporting is often delayed and inconsistent in format[3].

ADR is "any untoward medical occurrence that at any dose results in death, requires hospital admission or prolongation of existing hospital stay, results in persistent or significant disability/incapacity, or is life threatening."[4].

AIMS AND OBJETIVES

The aims and objectives of the study are:-

1. Identification and evaluation of the adverse drug reactions due to the anticancerous drugs in patients suffering from carcinoma.

2. Studying the clinical course of drug reactions.

3. Comparing the percentages of various drug reactions with those reported in literature.

4. Assessing the causality and preventability of the identified adverse drug reactions.

REVIEW OF LITERATURE

The goal of cancer treatment is first to eradicate the cancer. If this primary goal cannot be accomplished, the goal of cancer treatment shifts to palliation, the amelioration of symptoms, and preservation of quality of life while striving to extend life. The dictum primum non nocere[5] (means "first do no harm") is not necessarily the guiding principle of cancer therapy[6]. When cure of cancer is possible, cancer treatments may be undertaken despite the certainty of severe and perhaps life-threatening toxicities. Every cancer treatment has the potential to cause harm, and treatment may be given that produces toxicity with no benefit. The therapeutic index of many interventions is quite narrow, and most treatments are given to the point of toxicity. Conversely, when the clinical goal is palliation, careful attention to minimizing the toxicity of potentially toxic treatments becomes a significant goal. Irrespective of the clinical scenario, the guiding principle of cancer treatment should be primum succerrere, "first hasten to help"[6.] Radical surgical procedures, large-field hyper fractionated radiation therapy, high-dose chemotherapy, and maximum tolerable doses of cytokines such as interleukin (IL) 2 are all used in certain settings where 100% of the patients will experience toxicity and side effects from the intervention and only a fraction of the patients will experience benefit. One of the challenges of cancer treatment is to use the various treatment modalities alone and together in a fashion that maximizes the chances for patient benefit.

Cancer treatments are divided into four main types: surgery, radiation therapy (including photodynamic therapy), chemotherapy (including hormonal therapy and molecularly targeted therapy), and biologic therapy (including immunotherapy and gene therapy). The modalities are often used in combination, and agents in one category can act by several mechanisms. For example, cancer chemotherapy agents can induce differentiation, and antibodies (a form of immunotherapy) can be used to deliver radiation therapy. Surgery and radiation therapy are considered local treatments, though their effects can influence the behaviour of tumor at remote sites. Chemotherapy and biologic therapy are usually systemic treatments. Oncology, the study of tumors including treatment approaches, is a multidisciplinary effort with surgical, radiotherapy, and internal medicine–related areas of expertise[7].

4

Cancer agents have the potential for severe and occasionally fatal, adverse drug events. Many receive accelerated approval for use after small clinical trials, with adverse drug events being identified after further experience in the postmarketing clinical setting. Moreover, chemotherapy risks may be especially high in tertiary care settings whose patients frequently are subject to complex treatment protocols with high dosages, novel agents, or novel combinations of agents. The case of Betsy Lehman at the Dana-Farber Cancer Institute is a dramatic example of these risks. In 1994, as a participant in a clinical trial investigating a nonstandard schedule of cyclophosphamide, she received a fatal overdose[8]. Multiple system failures allowed the erroneous order to propagate over the course of four days.

HISTORY OF CHEMOTHERAPEUTIC DRUGS

The era of cancer chemotherapy began in the 1940s with the first use of nitrogen mustards and folic acid antagonist drugs[9].The beginnings of the modern era of cancer chemotherapy can be traced directly to the discovery of nitrogen mustard, a chemical warfare agent, as an effective treatment for cancer. Two pharmacologists, Louis S. Goodman and Alfred Gilman were recruited by the United States Department of Defense to investigate potential therapeutic applications of chemical warfare agents. Autopsy observations of people exposed to mustard gas had revealed profound lymphoid and myeloid suppression. Goodman and Gilman reasoned that this agent could be used to treat lymphoma, since lymphoma is a tumor of lymphoid cells. They first set up an animal model - they established lymphomas in mice and demonstrated they could treat them with mustard agents. Next, in collaboration with a thoracic surgeon, Gustav Linskog, they injected a related agent, mustine (the prototype nitrogen mustard anticancer chemotherapeutic), into a patient with non-hodgkin's lymphoma. They observed a dramatic reduction in the patient's tumour masses. Although this effect lasted only a few weeks, this was the first step to the realization that cancer could be treated by pharmacological agents (Goodman et al 1946).

Shortly after World War II, a second approach to drug therapy of cancer began. Sidney Farber, a pathologist at Harvard Medical School, studied the effects of folic acid on leukemia patients. Folic acid (citrovorum factor), a vitamin crucial for DNA metabolism[10] had been discovered by Lucy Wills, when she was working in India, in 1937. It seemed to stimulate the proliferation of acute lymphoblastic leukemia (ALL) cells when administered to children with this cancer. In one of the first examples of rational drug design (rather than accidental discovery), in collaboration with Harriett Kilte and Lederle Laboratories chemists, Farber used folate analogues. These analogues — first aminopterin and then amethopterin (now methotrexate) were antagonistic to folic acid, and blocked the function of folate-requiring enzymes. When administered to children with ALL in 1948, these agents became the first drugs to induce remission in children with ALL. Remissions were brief, but the principle was clear — antifolates could suppress proliferation of malignant cells, and could thereby re-establish normal bone-marrow function. It is worth noting that Farber met resistance to conducting his studies at a time when the commonly held medical belief was that leukemia was incurable, and that the children should be allowed to die in peace. Afterwards, Farber's 1948 report in the New England Journal of Medicine was met with incredulity and ridicule. In the same report he has amply appreciated the cooperation and guidance of the famous Biochemist, Dr. Y. SubbaRow (Director, Research Division, Lederle Labs, a division of American Cyanamid company, Pearl River, NY) who had synthesized and supplied the chemicals, Aminopterin and later Amithopterin for his clinical experiments. Remarkably, a decade later at the National Cancer Institute, Roy Hertz and Min Chiu Li discovered that the same methotrexate treatment alone could cure choriocarcinoma (1958), a germ-cell malignancy that originates in trophoblastic cells of the placenta. This was the first solid tumour to be cured by chemotherapy.

Joseph Burchenal, at Memorial Sloan-Kettering Cancer Center in New York, with Farber's help, started his own methotrexate study and found the same effects. He then decided to try and develop anti-metabolites in the same way as Farber, by making small changes in a metabolite needed by a cell to divide. With the help of George Hitchings and Gertrude Elion, two pharmaceutical chemists who were working at the Burroughs Wellcome Company in Tuckahoe, many purine analogues were tested, culminating in the Joseph Burchenal, at Memorial Sloan-Kettering Cancer Center in New York, with Farber's help, started his own methotrexate study and found the same effects. He then decided to try and develop anti-metabolites in the same way as Farber, by making small changes in a metabolite needed by a cell to divide. With the help of George Hitchings and Gertrude Elion, two pharmaceutical chemists who were working at the Burroughs Wellcome Company in Tuckahoe, many purine analogues were tested, culminating in the discovery of 6-mercaptopurine (6-MP), which was subsequently shown to be a highly active antileukemic drug.

The Eli Lilly natural products group found that alkaloids of the Madagascar periwinkle (Vinca rosea), originally discovered in a screen for anti-diabetic drugs, blocked proliferation of tumour cells. The antitumour effect of the vinca alkaloids (e.g. vincristine) was later shown to be due to their ability to inhibit microtubule polymerization, and therefore cell division.

The United States Congress created a National Cancer Chemotherapy Service Center (NCCSC) at the NCI in 1955 in response to early successes. This was the first federal programme to promote drug discovery for cancer - unlike now, most pharmaceutical companies were not yet interested in developing anticancer drugs. The NCCSC developed the methodologies and crucial tools (like cell lines and animal models) for chemotherapeutic development.

CANCER CHEMOTHERAPY: DRUG CLASSIFICATION AND MECHANISM OF ACTION[11]

CELL CYCLE EFFECTS OF MAJOR CLASSES OF ANTICANCER DRUGS:

CELL CYCLE – SPECIFIC (CCS) AGENTS	CELL CYCLE – NONSPECIFIC (CCNS) AGENTS
Antimetabolites (s phase)	**Alkylating agents**
Capecitabine	Altretamine
Cladribine	Bendamustine
Clofarabine	Busulfan
Cytarabine	Carmustine
Fludarabine	Chlorambucil
5-fluorouracil(5-FU)	Cyclophosphamide
Gemcitabine	Dacarbazine
6-mercaptopurine(6-MP)	Lomustine
Methotrexate(MTX)	Mechlorethamine
6-thioguanine (6-TG)	Melphalan
Epipodophyllotoxin (topoisomerase -2 inhibitor) (G_1-S phase)	Temozolomide
Etoposide	Thiotepa
Taxanes(M-phase)	**Anthracyclines**
Albumin bound paclitaxel	Daunorubicin
Docetaxel	Doxorubicin
Paclitaxel	Epirubicin
Vinca alkaloids(M phase)	Idarubicin
Vinblastine	Mitoxantrone
Vincristine	**Antitumor antibiotics**
Vinorelbine	Dactinomycin
Antimicrotubule inhibitor (M phase)	Mitomycin
Ixabipilone	**Camptothecins (topoisomerase 1 inhibitors)**
Antitumor antibiotics(G_2-M phase)	Irinotecan
Bleomycin	Topotecan
	Platinum analogs
	Carboplatin
	Cisplatin
	Oxaliplatin

ALKYLATING AGENTS AND PLATINUM ANALOGS: CLINICAL ACTIVITY AND TOXICITIES:

Alkylating Agent	Mechanism of action	Clinical applications	Acute toxicity	Delayed toxicity
Mechlorethamine	Forms DNA crosslinks, resulting in inhibition of DNA synthesis and function	Hodgkin's and non – hodgkin's lymphoma	Nausea & Vomiting	Moderate depression of peripheral blood count; excessive doses produce severe bone marrow depression with leucopenia, thrombocytopenia, and bleeding; alopecia and hemorrhagic cystitis occasionally occur with cyclophosphamide; cystitis can be prevented with adequate hydration ; busulfan is associated with skin pigmentation , pulmonary fibrosis, and adrenal insufficiency
Chlorambucil	Same as above	Cll and non-hodgkin's lymphoma	Nausea & vomiting	
Cyclophosphamide	Same as above	Breast cancer ,ovarian cancer, non – hodgkin's lymphoma,Cl l,soft tissue sarcoma, neuroblastom a, wilm's tumor,rhabdo myosarcoma	Nausea & vomiting	
Bendamustine	Same as above	Cll , non-hodgkin's lymphoma		

Alkylating Agent	Mechanism of action	Clinical applications	Acute toxicity	Delayed toxicity
Melphalan	Same as above	Multiple cancer ,breast cancer ,ovarian cancer	Nausea & vomiting	
Thiotepa	Same as above	Breast cancer , ovarian cancer, superficial bladder cancer	Nausea & vomiting	
Busulfan	Same as above	Cml	Nausea & vomiting	
Carmustine	Same as above	Brain cancer , hodgkin's and non-hodgkin's lymphoma	Nausea & vomiting	Myelosuppression; rarely: interstitial lung diseases and interstitial nephritis
Lomustine	Same as above	Brain cancer		
Altretamine	Same as above	Ovarian cancer	Nausea & vomiting	Myelosuppression , peripheral neuropathy ,flu-like syndrome
Temozolomide	Methylates DNA and inhibits DNA synthesis and function	Brain cancer and melanoma	Nausea & vomiting, headache and fatigue	Myelosuppression, mild elevation in liver function tests, photosensitivity
Procarbazine	Methylates DNA and inhibits DNA synthesis and function	Hodgkin's and non-hodgkin's , brain tumors	Central nervous system depression	Myelosuppression ,hypersensitivity reactions
Dacarbazine	Methylates DNA and inhibits DNA synthesis and function	Hodgkin's lymphoma,m elanoma and soft tissue sarcoma	Nausea & vomiting	Myelosuppression with neurotoxicity with neuropathy, ataxia,lethargy and confusion

Alkylating Agent	Mechanism of action	Clinical applications	Acute toxicity	Delayed toxicity
Cisplatin	Forms intrastrand and interstrand DNA cross-links; binding to nuclear and cytoplasmic proteins	Non-small cell and small cell lung cancer , breast cancer ,bladder cancer, gastroesophageal cancer, head and neck cancer, ovarian cancer ,germ cell cancer	Nausea and vomiting	Nephrotoxicity, peripheral sensory neuropathy, ototoxicity,nerve dysfunction
Carboplatin	Same as cisplatin	Non-small cell and small cell, breast cancer ,lung cancer, breast cancer, head and neck cancer, ovarian cancer ,bladder cancer	Nausea and vomiting	Myelosuppression; peripheral neuropathy ; renal toxicity, hepatic dysfunction
Oxaliplatin	Same as cisplatin	Colorectal cancer , gastroesophageal cancer , pancreatic cancer	Nausea and vomiting , laryngeal dysesthesias	Myelosuppression ,peripheral neuropathy , diarrhea

ANTIMETABOLITES: CLINICAL SPECTRUM OF ACTIVITY AND TOXICITIES:

Drug	Mechanism of action	Clinical applications	Toxicity
Capecitabine	Inhibits TS; incorporation of FUTP into RNA resulting in inhibition of DNA synthesis and function	Breast cancer ,colorectal cancer, gastroesophageal cancer, hepatocellular cancer,pancreatic cancer	Diarrhoea, hand-foot syndrome,myelosuppression,nausea and vomiting
5-Fluorouracil	Inhibits TS; incorporation of FUTP into RNA resulting in alteration in RNA processing;incorporation of FdUTP into DNA resulting in inhibition of DNA synthesis and function	Colorectal cancer, anal cancer, breast cancer, gastroesophageal cancer,head and cancer,hepatocellular cancer	Nausea, mucositis,diarrhea, bone marrow depression, neurotoxicity
Methotrexate	Inhibits DHFR;inhibits de novo purine nucleotide synthesis	Breast cancer ,head and neck cancer, osteogenic sarcoma,primary central nervous system lymphoma, non-hodgkin's lymphoma, bladder cancer , choriocarcinoma	Mucositis , diarrhea,myelosuppression with neutropenia and thrombocytopenia
Pemetrexed	Inhibits TS,DHFR, and purine nucleotide synthesis	Mesothelioma,non-small cell lung cancer ,	Myelosuppression ,skin rash ,mucositis diarrhea,fatigue
Cytarabine	Inhibits DNA chain elongation ,DNA synthesis and repair ;inhibits ribonucleotide reductase with reduced formation of dNTPs;incorporation of cytarabine triphosphate into DNA	AML,ALL,CML in blast crisis	Nausea ,vomiting ,myelosuppression, with neutropenia, and thrombocytopenia, cerebellar ataxia

Drug	Mechanism of action	Clinical applications	Toxicity
Gemcitabine	Inhibits DNA synthesis and repair ;inhibits ribonucleotiude reductase,with reduced formation of dNTPs; incorporation of gemcitabine triphosphate into DNA resulting in inhibition of DNA synthesis and function	Pancreatic cancer,bladder cancer,breast cancer,non-small cell lung cancer,ovarian cancer,non-hodgkin's lymphoma,soft tissue sarcoma	Nausea ,vomiting ,diarrhea, myelosupression
Fludarabine	Inhibits DNA synthesis and repair ;inhibits ribonucleotiude reductase,with reduced formation of dNTPs; resulting in inhibition of DNA; induction of apoptosis	Non-hodgkin's lymphoma,CLL	Myelosuppression, immunosuppression ,fever ,myalgias,arthralgias
Cladribine	Inhibits synthesis and repair,inhibits ribonucleotide reductase ;incorporation of cladiribine triphosphate into; induction of apoptosis	Hairy cell leukemia,CLL,non-hodgkin's lymphoma	Myelosuppression ,nausea , vomiting,immunosup pression
6-mercaptopurine	Inhibits de novo purine nucleotide synthesis; incorporation of triphosphate into RNA ;incorporation of triphosphate into DNA	AML	Myelosuppression ,immunosuppression ,hepatotoxicity
6-thioguanine	Same as above	ALL,AML	Same as above

NATURAL PRODUCT CANCER CHEMOTHERAPY DRUGS: CLINICAL ACTIVITY AND TOXICITIES:

Drug	Mechanism of Action	Clinical applications	Acute toxicity	Delayed toxicity
Bleomycin	Oxygen free radicals bind to DNA causing single – and double strand – DNA breaks	Hodgkin's and Non- Hodgkins lymphoma ,germ cell tumours , head and neck cancer	Allergic reactions, fever, hypotension	Skin toxicity,pulmonary fibrosis,mucositis alopecia
Daunorubicin	Oxygen free radicals bind to DNA causing single – and double strand – DNA breaks;inhibits topoisomerase -2	AML,ALL	Nausea ,fever, red urine (not hematuria)	Cardiotoxicity, alopecia, Myelo-suppression
Docetaxel	Inhibits mitosis	Breast cancer,non-small lung cancer,prostate cancer, gastric cancer,head and neck cancer ,ovarian cancer	Hypersensitivity	Neurotoxicity,fluid retention ,myelo-suppression
Doxorubicin	Oxygen free radicals bind to DNA causing single – and double strand – DNA breaks; intercalates DNA	Breast cancer, hodgkin's and non-hodgkin's lymphoma,soft tissue sarcoma,ovarian cancer,non-small cell cancer,thyroid cancer,wilm's tumour, neuroblastoma	Nausea , red urine	Cardiotoxicity ,myelo-suppression , stomatitis
Etoposide	Inhibits topoisomerase-2	Non-small cell lung cancer,small cell lung cancer,non-hodgkin's lymphoma,gastric cancer	Nausea, vomiting ,hypotension	Alopecia, myelo-suppression

Drug	Mechanism of Action	Clinical applications	Acute toxicity	Delayed toxicity
Idarubicin	Oxygen free radicals bind to DNA causing single – and double strand – DNA breaks; intercalates DNA	AML,ALL,CML	Nausea ,vomiting	Myelosuppression, mucositis, Cardiotoxicity
Irinotecan	Inhibits topoisomeraes -1	Colorectal cancer ,gastroesophageal cancer,non-small cell and small cell lung cancer	Diarrhea, nausea,vomiting	Myelosuppression
Mitomycin	Acts as an alkylating agent and and forms cross links with DNA; formation of oxygen free radical, which target DNA	Bladder cancer,breast cancer,gastric cancer , non-small cell lung cancer,head and neck cancer	Nausea ,vomiting	Myelosuppression ,mucositis,anorexia, fatigue,hemolytic uremic syndrome
Paclitaxel	Inhibits mitosis	Breast cancer, small cell and non-small cell lung cancer,ovarian cancer,gastroesophageal cancer, prostate cancer, head and neck cancer	Nausea, , vomiting, hypotension, arrhythmias, hypersensitivity	Myelosuppression ,peripheral neuropathy
Topotecan	Inhibits topoisomerase-1	Small cell lung cancer,ovarian cancer	Nausea , vomiting	Myelosuppression
Vinblastine	Inhibits mitosis	Breast cancer, hodgkin's and non-hodgkin's lymphoma, germ cell tumours, Kaposi's sarcoma	Nausea, vomiting	Myelosuppression, alopecia,mucositis , SIADH,vascular events

Drug	Mechanism of Action	Clinical applications	Acute toxicity	Delayed toxicity
Vincristine	Inhibits mitosis	ALL, hodgkin's and non-hodgkin's lymphoma, Rhabdomyo sarcoma, neuroblastoma,	None	Neurotoxicity ,peripheral neuropathy,para lytic ileus,myelosupp ression,alopecia , SIADH

MISCELLANEOUS ANTICANCER DRUGS: CLINICAL ACTIVITY AND TOXICITIES:

Drug	Mechanism of Action	Clinical Applications	Acute Toxicity	Delayed Toxicity
Arsenic trioxide	Induces differentiation of leukaemic cells by degrading the PML/RAR protein;induces apoptosis	Acute promyelocyti c leukaemia	Headache and light headedness	Fatigue, cardiac dysrrthmias,fever, dyspnoea
Asparaginase	Hydrolyzes circulating L-asparagine,resulti ng in rapid inhibition of protein synthesis	ALL	Nausea, fever ,allergy	Hepatotoxicity, bleeding, depression, pancreatitis, renal toxicity
Erlotinib	Inhibits EGFR tyrosine kinase leading to inhibition of EGFR signalling	Non-small cell lung cancer, Pancreatic cancer	Diarrhea	Skin rash,diarrhea, Anorexia,ILD
Imatinib	Inhibits Bcr-Abl tyrosine kinase and other receptor tyrosine kinases	CML,GIST, CLL	Nausea, Vomiting	Fluid retention,edema, Diarrhea,CCF

Drug	Mechanism of Action	Clinical Applications	Acute Toxicity	Delayed Toxicity
Cetuximab	Binds to EGFR And inhibits EGFR signaling; enhances responses to chemotherapy	Colorectal cancer, head and neck cancer, non small cell lung cancer	Infusion reaction	Skin rash, hypomagnesaemia, fatigue
Bevacizumab	Inhibits binding of VEGGF to VEGFR leading to inhibition of VEGF signaling;inhibits tumour vascular permeability but enhances tumour blood flow and drug delivery	Colorectal cancer ,breast cancer, non-small cell lung cancer	Hypertension, Infusion reaction	Thromboembolic events, proteinuria

TOXICITIES OF ALKYLATING AGENTS[9]

Bone Marrow Toxicity:

The alkylating agents differ in their patterns of antitumor activity and in the sites and severity of their side effects. Most cause dose-limiting toxicity to bone marrow elements, and to a lesser extent, intestinal mucosa. Most alkylating agents, including nitrogen mustard, melphalan, chlorambucil, cyclophosphamide, and ifosfamide, cause acute myelosuppression, with a nadir of the peripheral blood granulocyte count at 6 to 10 days and recovery in 14 to 21 days. Cyclophosphamide has lesser effects on peripheral blood platelet counts than do the other agents. Busulfan suppresses all blood elements, particularly stem cells, and may produce a prolonged and cumulative myelosuppression lasting months or even years. For this reason, it is used as a preparative regimen in allogenic bone marrow transplantation. Carmustine and other chloroethylnitrosoureas cause delayed and prolonged suppression of both platelets and granulocytes, reaching a nadir 4 to 6 weeks after drug administration and reversing slowly thereafter. Both cellular and humoral immunity are suppressed by alkylating agents, which have been used to treat various autoimmune diseases. Immunosuppression is reversible at doses used in most anticancer protocols.

Mucosal Toxicity:

In addition to effects on the hematopoietic system, alkylating agents are highly toxic to dividing mucosal cells, leading to oral mucosal ulceration and intestinal denudation. The mucosal effects are particularly significant in high-dose chemotherapy protocols associated with bone marrow reconstitution, as they predispose to bacterial sepsis arising from the gastrointestinal tract. In these protocols, cyclophosphamide, melphalan, and thiotepa have the advantage of causing less mucosal damage than the other agents. In high-dose protocols, however, a number of additional toxicities become limiting.

Neurotoxicity:

CNS toxicity is manifest in the form of nausea and vomiting, particularly after intravenous administration of nitrogen mustard or BCNU. Ifosfamide is the most neurotoxic of this class of agents, producing altered mental status, coma, generalized seizures, and cerebellar ataxia. These side effects have been linked to the release of chloroacetaldehyde from the phosphate-linked chloroethyl side chain of ifosfamide. High-dose busulfan may cause seizures; in addition, it accelerates the clearance of phenytoin, an antiseizure medication.

Other Organ Toxicities:
While mucosal and bone marrow toxicities occur predictably and acutely with conventional doses of these drugs, other organ toxicities may occur after prolonged or high-dose use; these effects can appear after months or years, and may be irreversible and even lethal. All alkylating agents have caused pulmonary fibrosis, usually several months after treatment. In high-dose regimens, particularly those employing busulfan or BCNU, vascular endothelial damage may precipitate veno-occlusive disease (VOD) of the liver, an often fatal side effect that is successfully reversed by the investigational drug defibrotide. The nitrosoureas and ifosfamide, after multiple cycles of therapy, may lead to renal failure. Cyclophosphamide and ifosfamide release a nephrotoxic and urotoxic metabolite, acrolein, which causes a severe hemorrhagic cystitis, a side effect that in high-dose regimens can be prevented by coadministration of 2-mercaptoethanesulfonate (mesna), which conjugates acrolein in urine. Ifosfamide in high doses for transplant causes a chronic, and often irreversible, renal toxicity. Proximal, and less commonly distal, tubules may be affected, with difficulties in Ca2+ and Mg2+ reabsorption, glycosuria, and renal tubular acidosis. Nephrotoxicity is correlated with the total dose of drug received and increases in frequency in children less than 5 years of age. The syndrome has been attributed to chloroacetaldehyde and/or acrolein excreted in the urine. The more unstable alkylating agents (particularly mechlorethamine and the nitrosoureas) have strong vesicant properties, damage veins with repeated use, and if extravasated, produce ulceration. Most alkylating agents cause alopecia.

Finally, all alkylating agents have toxic effects on the male and female reproductive systems, causing an often permanent amenorrhea, particularly in perimenopausal women, and an irreversible azoospermia in men.

Leukemogenesis:

As a class of drugs, the alkylating agents are highly leukemogenic. Acute nonlymphocytic leukemia, often associated with partial or total deletions of chromosome 5 or 7, peaks in incidence about 4 years after therapy and may affect up to 5% of patients treated on regimens containing alkylating drugs. It often is preceded by a period of neutropenia or anemia, and bone marrow morphology consistent with myelodysplasia. Melphalan, the nitrosoureas, and the methylating agent procarbazine have the greatest propensity to cause leukemia, while it is less common with cyclophosphamide.

ADVERSE EFFECTS OF ANTICANCEROUS DRUGS

The known adverse drug effects by anticancerous medications are broadly divided into:
1) Immediate
2) Delayed

IMMEDIATE ADVERSE DRUG REACTIONS

Among the immediate adverse effects the most common adverse drug reaction is the nausea, vomiting, fatigue and drowsiness, skin reactions, anorexia, mucositis and diarrhea closely follow the list[11].

Patterns of Chemotherapy induced nausea and vomiting (CINV) have also been defined based on symptom onset and duration, and include acute, delayed, breakthrough, refractory, and anticipatory CINV. Acute CINV begins within the first 24 hours after chemotherapy has started. Acute CINV can be further subdivided into nausea and vomiting occurring within the first 12 hours, and delayed acute nausea and vomiting occurring from 12 to 24 hours. Peak acuity usually occurs within six to seven hours of initiation of chemotherapy. Delayed nausea and vomiting develops more than 24 hours after chemotherapy initiation and may last for six to seven days. Carboplatin, cisplatin, cyclophosphamide, and doxorubicin are often associated with delayed nausea and vomiting. Due to the delay in symptoms from the time of chemotherapy infusion, delayed nausea and vomiting may be under-recognized. Breakthrough nausea and vomiting occurs despite anti-emetic prophylaxis and requires rescue medication. Refractory nausea and vomiting refers to symptoms that occur during subsequent treatment cycles after incomplete control in earlier cycles. Patients experiencing breakthrough nausea and vomiting are at risk for refractory nausea and vomiting and anticipatory nausea and vomiting. Anticipatory nausea and vomiting begins before chemotherapy, and is often associated with a history of poorly controlled acute and delayed CINV. Symptoms of anticipatory nausea and vomiting can be precipitated by taste, odor, sight, and anxiety, and this type of nausea may be difficult to treat[11].

Skin reactions

Table II. Classification of chemotherapeutic drugs according to their skin toxicity[12]

Non-aggressive cytostatics		Irritant cytostatics	Vesicant cytostatics	
Asparaginase	Bleomycin	Estramustine	Amsacrine	Mitomycin
Gemcytabine	Carmustine	Etoposide	Actinomycin C	Vinblastine
Fludarabine	Carboplatin	Fluorouracil	Daunorubicin	Vincristine
Cytarabine	Cyclophosphamide	Mitoxanthrone	Doxorubicin	Vindesine
Ifosfamide	Cisplatin	Paclitaxel	Epirubicin	Vinorelbine
Melphalan	Dacarbazine	Teniposide	Idarubicin	
Methotrexate	Docetaxel		Mechloretamine	

Cutaneous hypersensitivity reactions (Post-treatment skin reactions reported by cancer patients differ by race, not by treatment or expectations) Skin problems are among the common side effects of cancer treatment reported by patients, especially those undergoing radiation therapy for breast cancer and head and neck cancer. The combination of chemotherapy and radiation therapy has previously been reported to cause the worst skin reactions because chemotherapeutic drugs can induce radio sensitivity (Alley et al, 2002). The role that treatment regimen, skin pigmentation, and psychological factors play in the frequency of skin reactions experienced by cancer patients remains unclear. Possible prognostic factors for cancer treatment-related skin reactions should be identifiable by investigating the skin problems reported by cancer patients of different races in relation to their treatment type and pretreatment expectations. Skin pigmentation depends on the amount and distribution of a ubiquitous pigment known as melanin (Nielsen et al, 2006). Most reactions to standard chemotherapeutic agents are consistent with type 1 hypersensitivity, which is characterized by the rapid contraction of smooth muscle and dilation of capillaries, resulting in urticaria, rash, angioedema, bronchospasm, and hypotension[13].The skin of darkly pigmented individuals contains larger amounts of melanin, present as granules in melanocytes, resulting in a darker skin tone. Melanin protects human skin from ultraviolet (UV) and ionising radiation damage through its capacity to absorb light over a broad spectrum (Nielsen et al, 2006). Despite the protective capacity of melanin, both UV and ionising radiation can cause irreparable skin damage. Consequently, cancer patients have more severe radiation-induced skin reactions in sun-exposed areas of the skin, suggesting additive damage (Johansson et al, 2002)

Follicular rash is a side effect of chemotherapies and is one of the most consistent side effects with the HER1/EGFR inhibitors such as cetuximab, erlotinib, and gefitinib. The condition is also seen with some chemotherapies such as docetaxel, paclitaxel and epirubicin [14.]

Emetic risk of antineoplastic agents;[15,16]

High emetic risk	AC combination defined as either doxorubicin or epirubicin with cyclophosphamide Altretamine Carmustine (> 250 mg/m2) Cisplatin ($\geq$ 50 mg/m2) Cyclophosphamide (> 1,500 mg/m2) Dacarbazine Mechlorethamine Procarbazine (oral) Streptozocin
Moderate emetic risk	Aldesleukin (> 12–15 million units/m2)1 Amifostine (> 300 mg/m2) Arsenic trioxide Azacitidine Busulfan (> 4 mg/d) Carboplatin Carmustine ($\leq$ 250 mg/m2) Cisplatin (< 50 mg/m2) Cyclophosphamide ($\leq$ 1,500 mg/m2) Cyclophosphamide (oral) Cytarabine (> 1 g/m2) Dactinomycin Daunorubicin Doxorubicin Epirubicin Etoposide (oral) Idarubicin Ifosfamide Imatinib (oral)

	Irinotecan Lomustine Melphalan (> 50 mg/m2) Methotrexate (250 to > 1,000 mg/m2) Oxaliplatin (> 75 mg/m2) Temozolomide (oral) Vinorelbine (oral)
Low emetic risk	Amifostine ($\leq$ 300 mg) Bexarotene Capecitabine Cetuximab Cytarabine (low dose; [10]0–200 mg/m2) Docetaxel Doxorubicin (liposomal) Etoposide Fludarabine (oral) Fluorouracil Gemcitabine Methotrexate (> 50 mg/m2 to < 250 mg/m2) Mitomycin Mitoxantrone Paclitaxel Pemetrexed Topotecan1
Minimal emetic risk	Alemtuzumab Asparaginase Bevacizumab Bleomycin Chlorambucil (oral) Cladribine Gemtuzumab Hydroxyurea (oral) Melphalan (oral; low-dose) Methotrexate ($\leq$ 50 mg/m2) Rituximab Thioguanine (oral) Trastuzumab1 Valrubicin Vinblastine Vincristine Vinorelbine

Anorexia induced by chemotherapy[17]

The causes of anorexia in a patient suffering from cancer are various as the patient suffers weightloss syndrome and cachexia. Chemotherapy leads to mucositis and adds up to the cause. Anorexia varies in prevalence with different cancers and stage of disease (between 6% and 74%). It is more common in gastrointestinal malignancies and advanced diseases of gastric carcinomas (25% to 45% in patients receiving palliative care) and is often accompanied by malnourished states and cachexia[18].

DELAYED ADVERSE DRUG REACTIONS

Myelosuppression

Myelosuppression, the major dose-limiting toxicity of modern chemotherapy regimens. Myelosuppression is not only more common in the elderly but also more severe, resulting in longer hospital stays and higher inpatient mortality. The risk of neutropenia and its complications, including death, is highest in the early cycles of chemotherapy. Because of this risk and the potential for better outcomes, prophylaxis with a colony-stimulating factor beginning in the first cycle should be considered in elderly patients .The influence of age on the risk of chemotherapy-induced anemia has received little attention, despite the prevalence of this condition in older patients with cancer[19]. Myelosuppression induces release of growth factors that stimulates extra cell divisions in the proliferating compartments and shortens the time at which mature cells reach the circulation[20].

Mucosal Toxicity

In addition to effects on the hematopoietic system, alkylating agents are highly toxic to dividing mucosal cells, leading to oral mucosal ulceration and intestinal denudation[21]. The mucosal effects are particularly significant in high-dose chemotherapy protocols associated with bone marrow reconstitution, as they predispose to bacterial sepsis arising from the gastrointestinal tract. In these protocols, cyclophosphamide, melphalan, and thiotepa have the advantage of causing less mucosal damage than the other agents. In high-dose protocols, however, a number of additional toxicities become limiting[9]. Mucositis is an inflammatory reaction that affects the entire gastrointestinal tract, although with a greater involvement of the oropharyngeal area. Clinically it appears between approximately the fifth and seventh day from the start of chemotherapy, the lesions being located fundamentally in the non-keratinized oral mucosa[22,23].

The manifestations of mucositis rank from 0 to IV Grade 0: no symptoms; Grade I: painless ulcers, erythema or mild soreness; Grade II: painful erythema, edema or ulcers, but the patient can eat solid meal; Grade III: painful erythema, edema or ulcers, and the patient cannot eat solid meal; Grade IV: requires parenteral or enteral support[24].

Neurologic complications of cancer chemotherapy
Some are dose-related, while others may arise in the presence of specific risk factors. Lastly, some are idiosyncratic. The most common effect of chemotherapy on the PNS is a sensory neuropathy. Lhermitte's syndrome[25,26], is sometimes seen, suggesting central involvement. Importantly, patients with pre-existing neuropathies are at increased risk of severe neurotoxicity.

Chemotherapy may affect the central nervous system in a number of ways, such as acute encephalopathy, that is often reversible, or a chronic CNS toxicity that may be additive with radiotherapy, such as with methotrexate or intra-arterial chemotherapy. Focal disorders include cerebellar syndromes, such as with high dose cytarabine. Levamisole when combined with 5-FU may cause a multifocal leucoencephalopathy, with enhancing subcortical white matter lesions that can be mistaken for cerebral metastases. Transverse myelopathy may occur with intrathecal therapy, or as mentioned above, Lhermitte's phenomenon may be seen with oxaliplatin. Autonomic dysfunction can cause constipation, and even postural hypotension. The acute neurotoxicity seen with oxaliplatin is characterised by electrophysiologic evidence motor nerve hyperexcitability. Cisplatinum encephalopathy is commonly associated with hypomagnesaemia, which also should be treated, and seizure control is important[26].

Neurotoxicity
CNS toxicity is manifest in the form of nausea and vomiting, particularly after intravenous administration of nitrogen mustard or BCNU. Ifosfamide is the most neurotoxic of this class of agents, producing altered mental status, coma, generalized seizures, and cerebellar ataxia. These side effects have been linked to the release of chloroacetaldehyde from the phosphate-linked chloroethyl side chain of ifosfamide. High-dose busulfan may cause seizures; in addition, it accelerates the clearance of phenytoin, an antiseizure medication[9].

Leukemogenesis
As a class of drugs, the alkylating agents are highly leukemogenic[9]. Acute nonlymphocytic leukemia, often associated with partial or total deletions of chromosome 5 or 7, and balanced translocations involving chromosomes 11 and 23

after exposure to topoisomerase II inhibitors [27] peaks in incidence about 4 years after therapy and may affect up to 5% of patients treated on regimens containing alkylating drugs (Levine and Bloomfield, 1992)[9]. As the evidence base for alkylating agents in oncology practice strengthened, t-AML was reported after treatment for a variety of hematological malignancies and solid tumors. The subsequent introduction of topoisomerase II inhibitors into oncology practice was quickly followed by reports of t-AML in both hematological malignancies and breast cancer[28], the time course to AML after exposure to alkylating agents was typically five or more years and was frequently associated with a preexisting myelodysplastic syndrome [29]. In contrast, t-AML after topoisomerase II inhibitors was associated with a latent period of 2–3 years, typically without a pre-existing myelodysplastic syndrome [28].

Other Organ Toxicities

All alkylating agents have caused pulmonary fibrosis, usually several months after treatment. In high-dose regimens, particularly those employing busulfan or BCNU, vascular endothelial damage may precipitate veno-occlusive disease (VOD) of the liver[9]. The nitrosoureas[30] and ifosfamide[31], after multiple cycles of therapy, may lead to renal failure[9]. Cyclophosphamide[32] and ifosfamide release a nephrotoxic and urotoxic metabolite, acrolein[33], which causes a severe hemorrhagic cystitis. Most alkylating agents cause alopecia. Finally, all alkylating agents have toxic effects on the male and female reproductive systems, causing an often permanent amenorrhea, particularly in perimenopausal women, and an irreversible azoospermia in men.

Cardiotoxicity is a potential side effect of few chemotherapeutic agents. The anthracycline class of cytotoxic antibiotics is the most famous, but other chemotherapeutic agents can also cause serious cardiotoxicity and are not so well recognised. Examples include cyclophosphamide, ifosfamide, mitomycin and fluorouracil[34].Cardiotoxicity of cancer chemotherapeutics is a problem for patients of all ages, but it increases with age. Toxicity can also develop months after the last chemotherapy dose, and late reactions can be seen years later when they present as new-onset cardiomyopathy, often in patients who were treated for childhood neoplasms[35].

29

PHARMACOLOGICAL CONSIDERATIONS

During past decades pharmacological drug development has made it quite clear that there is a need for new and more active drugs in cancer chemotherapy. The strategies used so far for the development of cytotoxic drugs have been based on empirical observations, rational drug design based on suitable targets as evident from research in cellular biochemistry, synthesis of analogs to already known active drugs and the use of laboratory systems for screening of cytotoxic properties among chemicals available [36]. Drug development has relied on the testing of the drug against various tumour cell lines in the laboratory followed by evaluation in tumour-bearing mice. Following this preclinical development, the new drugs are tested at increasing doses in cancer patients with the aim to define the optimal dose to be used in larger clinical studies to define the antitumour activity. A bearing principle in the development process for new cytotoxic drugs is the hope that there may perhaps be targets in tumour cells that are not present in normal cells and the exploitation of which may confer a more advantageous therapeutic index for cytotoxic drugs. The finding of such targets may well be related to the research on the mechanisms regulating apoptosis and cell cycle progression. However, there are also several other putative targets for new drugs. Among these are tumour-specific properties in the cell signal transmission system, cell membrane composition, angiogenesis, telomerase and matrix interaction[36].

With respect to the process of drug development there is reason to believe that it will become more efficient. By the addition of laboratory testing systems with good correlation to activity in the patients, the preclinical part of new drug development may become more rapid and efficient than so far. Besides rational drug design, there will probably also be space in the future for progress in drug development based on analog-synthesis, unprejudiced drug screening and exploitation of serendipitous findings. The paradigm of individualized drug therapy based on a person's unique genetic make-up is especially desirable in the field of oncology, where the therapeutic index is often narrow and the consequences of drug toxicity can be life threatening. Generally, anticancer agents are administered at the maximally tolerated dose[37], as defined for a large population, with an expectation that approximately a third of patients will have unacceptable toxicity. Polymorphisms that affect drug clearance often lead to recognizable clinical events, such as myelosuppression or neurotoxicity. Thus, if clinicians could better predict which individuals are at the greatest risk of suffering chemotherapy-related toxicities, then the overall care of cancer patients could be greatly impacted with patient-specific dose modifications, optimization of treatment choice (when several equivalent therapies exist), or avoidance of a therapy when toxicity risks outweigh potential benefits. More important is the ability to predict those patients at greatest risk for nonresponse to specific treatment, as modifying their therapeutic regimen could be highly beneficial. In addition to environmental influences, variation in the genetic constitution between individuals will have a major impact on drug activity. Single-nucleotide polymorphisms (SNPs) account for over 90% of genetic variation in the human genome. The remainder of the variation is caused by insertions and deletions (indels), tandem repeats and microsatellites. With the completion of the human genome project, there has been an explosion in the discovery, characterisation and validation of genetic variation. Over 1.42 million SNPs were initially identified through the human genome project (Sachidanandam et al, 2001), and a goldmine of SNP information is now readily accessible via publicly available databases (Marsh et al, 2002). In addition, affordable, high throughput genotyping technologies are now available, including Pyrosequencing, FP-TDI, MALDI-TOF and SNP chips, making pretreatment genotyping a real possibility[38].

VARIOUS SCALES USED IN ADR MONITIRING

Causality assessment is the method by which the extent of relationship between a drug and a suspected reaction is established. Currently wide varieties of causality assessment scales exist, to attribute clinical events to drugs in individual patients or in case reports, each with their own advantages and limitations.

These scales include

- ❖ Karch & Lasagna scale
- ❖ Naranjo's scale
- ❖ WHO probability scale
- ❖ Spanish quantitative imputation scale
- ❖ Kramer's scale
- ❖ Jones scale
- ❖ European ABO system
- ❖ Bayesian system.

The Naranjo's scale and the WHO scale of assessment are the most commonly used scales. The Naranjo algorithm can be used to assess the likelihood that a change in clinical status is the result of an ADR rather than the result of other factors such as progression of disease. Answer each of the ten items in the assessment and enter the value of the answer in the column labelled Score. Sum the scores of the ten items to determine the total score, and apply the interpretation rules that appear at the bottom of the page.

NARANJO ALGORITHM FOR ADR CAUSALITY ASSESSMENTM FOR ADR[39]:

Naranjo Algorithm for ADR Causality Assessment	Yes	No	Don't Know	Score
1. Are there previous conclusive reports of this reaction?	+1	0	0	____
2. Did the adverse event appear after the suspect drug was administered?	+2	-1	0	____
3. Did the adverse reaction improve when the drug was discontinued?	+1	0	0	____
4. Did the adverse reaction reappear when the drug was readministered?	+2	-1	0	____
5. Are there alternate causes that on their own could have caused the reaction?	-1	+2	0	____
6. Did the reaction appear when a placebo was given?	-1	+1	0	____
7. Was the drug detected in the blood (or other fluids) in concentrations known to be toxic?	+1	0	0	____
8. Was the reaction more severe when the dose was increased or less severe when decreased?	+1	0	0	____
9. Did the patient have a similar reaction to the same or similar drugs in any previous exposure?	+1	0	0	____
10. Was the adverse event confirmed by any objective evidence?	+1	0	0	____
			Total score =	____

Interpretation of the Total Score

Total scores of 9 or more mean that an ADR is highly probable.

Scores from 5 to 8 mean that an ADR is probable.

Scores from 1 to 4 that an ADR is possible.

Scores of zero or less mean that an ADR is doubtful.

WHO SCALE OF ASSESSMENT[40]

1.CERTAIN	A clinical event, including laboratory test abnormality, occurring in a plausible time relationship to drug administration, and which cannot be explained by concurrent disease or other drugs or chemicals. The response to withdrawal of the drug (dechallenge) should be clinically plausible. The event must be definitive pharmacologically or phenomenologically, using a satisfactory rechallenge procedure if necessary.
2.PROBABLE/ LIKELY	A clinical event, including laboratory test abnormality, with a reasonable time sequence to administration of the drug, unlikely to be attributed to concurrent disease or other drugs or chemicals, and which follows a clinically reasonable response on withdrawal (dechallenge). Rechallenge information is not required to fulfil this definition.ical event, including laboratory test abnormality, with a reasonable time sequence to administration of the drug, unlikely to be attributed to concurrent disease or other drugs or chemicals, and which follows a clinically reasonable response on withdrawal (dechallenge). Rechallenge information is not required to fulfil this definition.
3.POSSIBLE	A clinical event, including laboratory test abnormality, with a reasonable time sequence to administration of the drug, but which could also be explained by concurrent disease or other drugs or chemicals. Information on drug withdrawal may be lacking or unclear.
4.UNLIKELY	A clinical event, including laboratory test abnormality, with a temporal relationship to drug administration which makes a causal relationship improbable, and in which other drugs, chemicals or underlying disease provide plausible explanations.
5.CONDITIONAL/ UNCLASSIFIED	A clinical event, including laboratory test abnormality, reported as an adverse reaction, about which more data is essential for a proper assessment or the additional data are under examination.
6.UNASSESSIBLE/ UNCLASSIFIABLE	A report suggesting an adverse reaction which cannot be judged because information is insufficient or contradictory, and which cannot be supplemented or verified.

PROBLEMS WITH ALGORITHMS[39]

Although algorithms have better reproducibility than clinical judgment in rating ADRs, clinical judgment with its low inter- and intra-rater agreement still plays a big part in the identification and rating of potential ADRs by an algorithm. This is because the answers to some of the questions in the algorithm may be affected by clinical judgment. More importantly the first step in ADR identification depends on a clinical judgment, i.e. the decision that this might be an ADR and so deserves further assessment using an algorithm. Further problems include that the questions in an algorithm are often weighted, these weights are arbitrarily assigned based on their perceived importance and vary between algorithms. This qualitative assigning of weights means that algorithms are unable to truly determine the probability of the ADR causality. Even though algorithms have been shown to be more reproducible than clinical judgment alone, the validity of the measure must also be considered. The fact that the algorithms agree well with each other does not mean that they are right. Studies have looked at the validity of algorithms, by comparing the category of causality that they produce to the decision on causality decided by a group of experts in the field. This is not a true test of the validity of an assessment system, as this testing cannot work as for as the majority of ADRs, no true "Gold Standard" exists. Further problems include the idea that most include questions on dechallenge/ rechallenge, and the rechallenge often does not occur in the "real world" of clinical practice. This might not occur for a number of reasons, for many serious ADRs rechallenge might be considered unethical, since it may pose a considerable risk to the patient. Also for many lesser potential ADRs using a different drug rather than undergoing the rechallenge may well be deemed an easier and simpler option by the clinician. Even if the clinician is willing to consider rechallenge to strengthen the probability of causality for an ADR, the patients themselves will often refuse such a rechallenge. Without a rechallenge it is difficult with most of these algorithms for causality to be graded more than "possible". Algorithms depend on a YES/NO answer to individual questions, this is not always easy, sometimes a "maybe" might be more appropriate. So in away algorithms may simply replace honesty with pragmatism. Lastly there are a great number of ADRs in a number of different body systems, so a single standardized assessment tool may not be ideal for such a diversity of possible presentations.

Determining if an adverse event is caused by a certain drug with reasonable certainty is a difficult part of ADRs' evaluation, but it is essential for proper clinical decisions .The aim of the causality assessment is to establish a level of probability regarding the suspicion that a certain drug is responsible for an adverse event. According to the most widely used with or without score algorithms, ADRs can be "certain", "probable/likely", "possible" and "unlikely/doubtful". The WHO-UMC developed a causality system which takes into account the clinical-pharmacological aspects, whereas previous knowledge of the ADR plays a less prominent role[41].

In order to take appropriate initiatives towards the management of the ADR, it is necessary to study the severity of the ADRs. Hartwig scale (Hartwig et al, 1992) is widely used for the purpose. This scale categorizes the reported adverse drug reactions into different levels as mild, moderate or severe. In Mild (Level 1) the ADR requires no change in the treatment with the suspected drug and Mild (Level 2) the ADR requires that the suspected drug be withheld, discontinued or otherwise changed. No antidote or other treatment is required, and there is no increase in lenght of stay. In Moderate (Level 3) the ADR requires that the suspected drug be withheld, discontinued or otherwise changed, and/ or an antidote or other treatment is required with no increase in length of stay. Moderate [Level 4 (a)] is any level 3 ADR that increases the length of stay by at least one day and in Moderate [Level 4 (b)] the ADR is the reason for admission. The Severe (Level 5) is any level 4 ADR that requires intensive medical care, Severe (Level 6) is the ADR causing parmanent harm to the patient and Severe (Level 7) being the ADR either directly or indirectly leading to the death of the patient[42].

Preventable adverse drug reaction was defined according to Schumock and Thornton (1992) as ADR which was preventable or avoidable. The original Schumock-Thornton algorithm assesses prescribing errors, which can be defined as dosing errors or therapeutic errors, such as medication not indicated (based on patient history), medication contraindicated, recorded medication allergies, drug-drug interaction (included only if the interaction is inadequately monitored or if the medication involved in the interaction may never be combined [absolute contraindication and indication for the combination]), inadequate monitoring of therapy, therapeutic duplication medication, and under prescribing (defined as an essential medicine not being prescribed).The algorithm was expanded to include dispensing errors (errors at the dispensing stage in the pharmacy) and administration errors (errors when administering medicate on to the patient either by caretakers or by the patient, eg, nonadherence to the medication regimen). If the assessments of the pharmacists disagreed, they met to reach consensus (2.5% of the cases for the causality assessment and 26% of the cases for the preventability assessment)[43].

Modified Schumock[44] and thornton[45] scale for preventability of adverse drug reaction assessment[46].

Criteria for determining preventability of an adverse drug reaction (ADR)[46]
Section A
Answering "yes" to one or more of the following implies that an
ADR is DEFINITELY preventable
1. Was there a history of allergy or previous reactions to the drug?
2. Was the drug involved inappropriate for the patient's clinical condition?
3. Was the dose, route, or frequency of administration inappropriate for the patient's age, weight, or disease state?
If answers are all negative to the above, then proceed to Section B
Section B
Answering "yes" to one or more of the following implies that an
ADR is PROBABLY preventable
1. Was required therapeutic drug monitoring or other necessary laboratory tests not performed?
2. Was a documented drug interaction involved in the ADR?
3. Was poor compliance involved in the ADR?
4. Was a preventative measure not administered to the patient?
5. If a preventative measure was administered, was it inadequate and/or inappropriate? Answer 'NO' if this question is nonapplicable
If answers are all negative to the above, then proceed to Section C.
Section C
The ADR is NOT preventable

MATERIALS AND METHODS

This study was undertaken in the wards and outpatient Departments of Goa Medical College, Bambolim, Goa, with the approval of the concerned ethical committee. Study involved patients treated on chemotherapy and diagnosed with cancer. The duration of study is of one year from 1-7-2009 to 1-7-2010.

PATIENT SELECTION:

Patients diagnosed as having a carcinoma using histological and various clinical methods formed the study sample. Inpatients as well as outpatients coming for regular follow-ups were a part of this study.

INCLUSION CRITERIA:

Patients of either gender, irrespective of age and diagnosed as carcinoma and receiving chemotherapy were included in the study.

EXCLUSION CRETERIA:

1) Patients exclusively on radiotherapy were not the part of study
2) Patients receiving chemotherapeutic medications for ailments other than carcinoma were excluded from the study.

STUDY DESIGN:

This study is based on prospective observational design with patients prescribed for anticancer chemotherapy. A detailed medication history and general physical examination was done. The laboratory reports were assessed and detailed history of illness was taken. Naranjo algorithm was the standard scale used to assess the causality of the adverse drug reactions. Modified Schumock-Thornton algorithm was used to assess the preventability of the adverse drug reactions.

Naranjo algorithm to assess the causality used in our study.

Naranjo Algorithm for ADR Causality Assessment	Yes	No	Don't Know	Score
1. Are there previous conclusive reports of this reaction?	+1	0	0	_____
2. Did the adverse event appear after the suspect drug was administered?	+2	-1	0	_____
3. Did the adverse reaction improve when the drug was discontinued?	+1	0	0	_____
4. Did the adverse reaction reappear when the drug was readministered?	+2	-1	0	_____
5. Are there alternate causes that on their own could have caused the reaction?	-1	+2	0	_____
6. Did the reaction appear when a placebo was given?	-1	+1	0	_____
7. Was the drug detected in the blood (or other fluids) in concentrations known to be toxic?	+1	0	0	_____
8. Was the reaction more severe when the dose was increased or less severe when decreased?	+1	0	0	_____
9. Did the patient have a similar reaction to the same or similar drugs in any previous exposure?	+1	0	0	_____
10. Was the adverse event confirmed by any objective evidence?	+1	0	0	_____
			Total score =	_____

Interpretation of the Total Score

Total scores of 9 or more mean that an ADR is highly probable.

Scores from 5 to 8 mean that an ADR is probable.

Scores from 1 to 4 that an ADR is possible.

Scores of zero or less mean that an ADR is doubtful.

Following Modified Schumock-Thornton algorithm was used to assess the preventability of the adverse drug reactions in the present study.

Criteria for determining preventability of an adverse drug reaction (ADR)
Section A
Answering "yes" to one or more of the following implies that an
ADR is DEFINITELY preventable
1. Was there a history of allergy or previous reactions to the drug?
2. Was the drug involved inappropriate for the patient's clinical condition?
3. Was the dose, route, or frequency of administration inappropriate for the patient's age, weight, or disease state?
If answers are all negative to the above, then proceed to Section B
Section B
Answering "yes" to one or more of the following implies that an
ADR is PROBABLY preventable
1. Was required therapeutic drug monitoring or other necessary laboratory tests not performed?
2. Was a documented drug interaction involved in the ADR?
3. Was poor compliance involved in the ADR?
4. Was a preventative measure not administered to the patient?
5. If a preventative measure was administered, was it inadequate and/or inappropriate? Answer 'NO' if this question is nonapplicable
If answers are all negative to the above, then proceed to Section C.
Section C
The ADR is NOT preventable

RESULTS

The results of the study were based on the adverse drug profile of the various regimens used in the tertiary care centre that is Goa Medical College and Hospital for various types of carcinoma seen in the population. The main regimens used were the FEC regimen[47,48] (Fluorouracil (5FU), epirubicin and cyclophosphamide) for the breast cancer and cisplatin/cyclophosphamide or carboplatin/paclitaxel regimen for the ovarian cancer[49,50]. The general trend of adverse drug effects reported in the literature has already been mentioned. The findings in the study depicting the side effects of the regimen or the drugs used have been shown as a master chart.

The general trend of adverse drug effects reported in the literature has already been mentioned. The findings in the study depicting the side effects of the regimen or the drugs used have been shown as a master chart. Master chart shows the name, age, sex, diagnosis, treatment given, adverse drug reactions, hospital number, associated drugs, date of admission.

The naranjo algorithm scale for assessing adverse drug reactions was used to assess the severity of the reaction. Among the 202 patients observed in the study, the percentage of females was 66% (133) and males was 34% (69),[fig.1,table 1], total number of adverse drug reactions were 891[master chart] as observed by bed to bed examination by resident doctors examination with the help of lab diagnosis.

Almost 53 percent of the adverse drug reactions according to naranjo algorithm were categorized as "probable" with score ranging from 5-8 and 47 percent were categorized as "possible" with score ranging from 1-4. Assessment of preventability of the adverse drug reaction was done based on modified schumock and thornton scale[51]. Most of the adverse drug reactions belonged to the category "not preventable" However the more common reactions like nausea and vomiting belonged to the category of "preventable" adverse drug reactions.

Table 1: Showing the distribution of male and female patients in the study.

Number of patients	Male	Female
202	69	133

Fig. 1: Bar chart showing the distribution of female and male patients in the study.

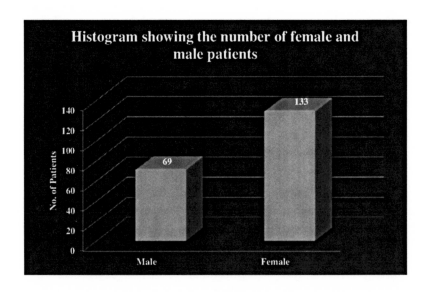

Table 2: Showing the age distribution of the patients.

Age group	Number of patients
0 – 9	7
10 – 19	6
20 – 29	13
30 – 39	23
40 – 49	38
50 – 59	62
60 – 69	39
70 – 79	13
80 – 89	1

Fig.2: Bar graph showing the prevalence of patients in different age groups receiving chemotherapy.

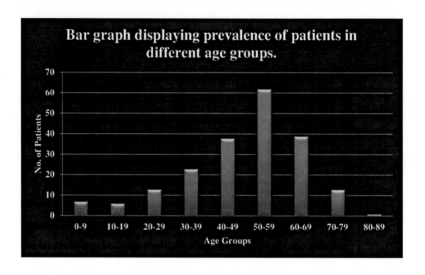

Bar graph displaying prevalence of patients in different age groups.

The prevalence of patients receiving chemotherapy mostly belonged to the age group between 50 and 59 years, among the patients under study [fig.2, table 2, fig.3]. The male to female ratio was 1:1.9. The prevalence of various cancers that were observed in the study is shown below in the following graphs and pie charts. The study revealed 35% (70) of the patients suffered breast carcinoma in various stages and types, followed by 15% of patients (30) suffered gastrointestinal carcinoma. The number of patients who suffered carcinoma of ovary is 25 accounting to 12% of the population under study. The patients suffering lung carcinoma was 8% accounting to 16 patients of the total 202 patients. Hematological carcinomas accounted for 12 patients forming 6% of total population under study. Number of patients suffering oral cavity cancers is 9 accounting to 4 percent of the population of patients in our study. Brain cancers accounted to approximately 4 percent of the population under study and the number of patients observed is 8. Total number of patients suffering carcinoma of larynx is 9 which are observed in 4 percent of the patients. A total of 3 patients suffered carcinoma of cervix which is observed in approximately 2 percent of population. Rest of the patients yet not stated above were those suffering -Primitive neuroectodermal tumor (PNET), Hodgkins disease, Non Hodgkins disease, retinoblastoma, seminoma of testis and wilm's tumor[fig.4,table-3,fig.5].

Fig. 3: Pie diagram displays percentage prevalence of patients in different age group receiving chemotherapy.

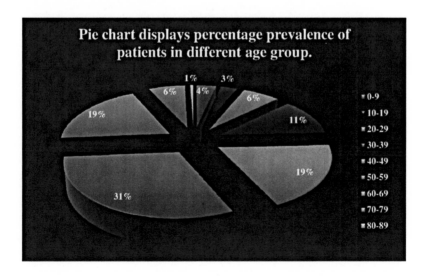

Fig. 4: Pie chart showing percentage of different types of carcinomas observed in the study.

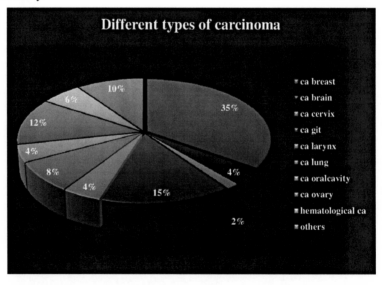

Table 3: Showing the number of patients diagnosed with various carcinomas in the study.

Carcinoma	Number of patients
Ca breast	70
Ca brain	8
Ca cervix	3
Ca GIT	30
Ca larynx	9
Ca lung	16
Ca oral cavity	9
Ca ovary	25
Hematological Ca	12
Others	20

Fig. 5: Displaying the number of patients diagnosed with respective carcinomas.

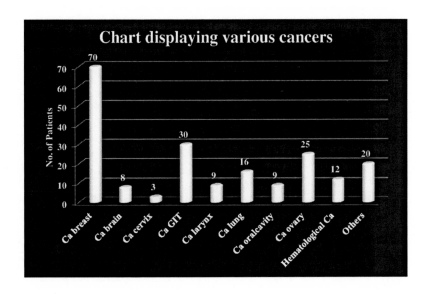

Table 4: Showing the number of patients prescribed with various types of chemotherapeutic drugs.

Chemotherapeutics used	Number of patients
Alkylating agents	167
Antimatabolites	133
Natural products	80
antibiotics	77
miscellaneous	46

Fig. 6: Pie chart shows percentage of various types of chemotherapeutic drugs used in the study.

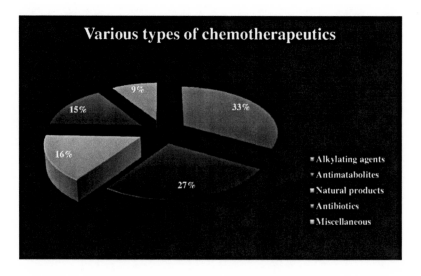

Among the various chemotherapeutics used in the study 33 percent of the drugs administered were alkylating agents among which cyclophosphamide is the most commonly used with cisplatin , carboplatin , oxaliplatin and temozolomide in the descending order of use. Dacarbazine, chlorambucil and mechlorethamine were also prescribed to the patients under study. The use of antimetabolites in the study as observed was 27 percent among the total drug therapy which included 5-fluorouracil, capecitabine, gemcitabine and methotrexate in descending order of use. Cladribine, 6-mercaptopurine, 6-thioguanine and Cytarabine are also administred to the patients Natural products (excluding anticancer antibiotics) in the cancer therapy include docetaxel, etoposide, irinotecan, paclitaxel, vincristine and vinblastine were responsible for 16% of total anticancerous chemotherapeutic drugs. Among this group paclitaxel was more commonly used in the present study viz; to those patients who were diagnosed as suffering from ovarian carcinomas. Anticancer antibiotics formed 15 percent of advice on the prescription in inpatient department (IPD) charts of patients in the present study. Most commonly used antibiotics was epirubicin commonly in the FEC regimen [Fluorouracil (5FU), epirubicin and cyclophosphamide] used in the treatment of breast cancers. In the miscellaneous group the most commonly used drugs are the monoclonal antibodies like rituximab and cetuximab, the list also includes lapatinib, imatinib, and asparagenase. The percentage of prescription of miscellaneous agents is 9 percent. Adjuvant chemotherapy formed the backbone of the study which was administered to a total of 188 patients and this accounted to the administration of the adjuvant chemotherapy to 94 percent of patients in our study while chemotherapy alone was administered to 6 percent of the people in the study [fig.6, table.4, fig.7].

Fig. 7: Bar graph showing various chemotherapeutics in x-axis and number of patients in y-axis.

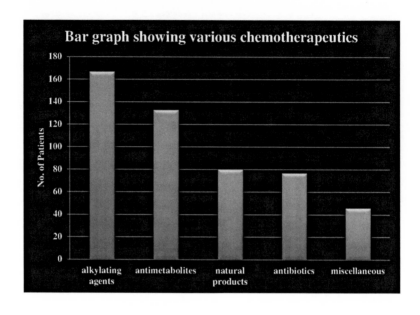

Fig. 8: Pie chart showing the percentage prevalence of different adverse drug reactions in different age groups.

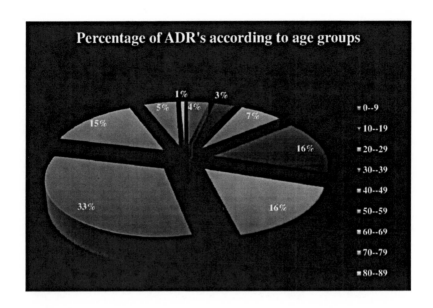

Table 5: Showing percentage prevalence of adverse drug reactions according to the age groups.

Age group	Percentage of ADR's in different age group
0 – 9	3.55
10 – 19	3.44
20 – 29	7.11
30 – 39	15.88
40 – 49	16.33
50 – 59	32.44
60 – 69	15.22
70 – 79	5.44
80 – 89	0.59

Fig. 9: Bar graph showing the percentage prevalence of different adverse drug reactions in different age groups.

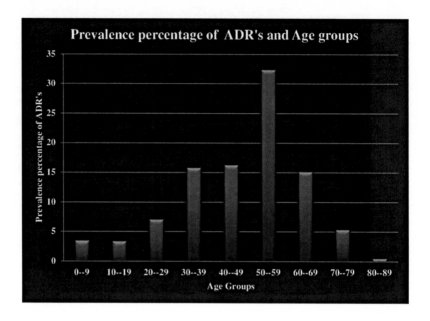

The maximum percentage prevalence of adverse drug reactions occurred in the age group between 50 and 59 years which accounted to 33 percent of patients in the study. The percentage prevalence of patients increased gradually forming a peak at the age group (in years) of 50-59 and then had a decline[fig.8,table.5,fig.9]. However, the incidence of cancers is more common in the old age. Adverse drug reactions according to the age group is increasing till the age of 6th decade in the present study and then the decline in the number of adverse drug reactions in the further age group is observed.

Fig. 10: Pie chart displaying various adverse drug reactions in percentage.

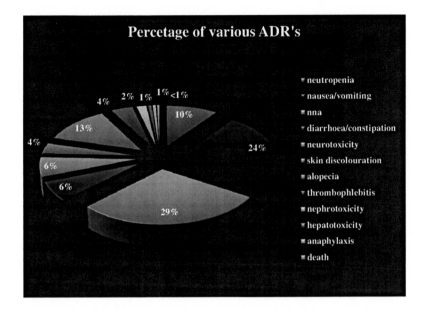

Among the various adverse drug reactions assessed in the study, hematological toxicity is the most common to be observed. Among all the adverse drug reactions 29 percent of them were normocytic normochromic anaemia. The study revealed that 10 percent of patients suffered neutropenia.

Table 6: Showing the number of patients and different adverse drug reactions.

ADR's	Number of patients
Neutropenia	58
Nausea/vomiting	144
Nna	170
Diarrhoea/constipation	38
Neurotoxicity	39
Skin discolouration	22
Alopecia	75
Thrombophlebitis	25
Nephrotoxicity	11
Hepatotoxicity	4
Anaphylaxis	4
Death	2

The next adverse drug reaction observed in the study was nausea/vomiting which formed 24 percent of total number of adverse drug reactions. Alopecia was observed in 13 percent of patients. However, the number of patients suffering total baldness was not more. Baldness was observed more commonly with the patients undergoing treatment with FEC regimen.

Neurotoxicity was observed in 6 percent of the adverse drug reactions in the study. The various features representing neurotoxicity associated with chemotherapy include nausea/vomiting, peripheral neuropathies, abdominal neuropathies, Loss of vibration sense, paraesthesia, ataxia and ototoxicity.

Skin discoloration is observed in 6 percent of the patients with various adverse drug reactions. Various causes associated with skin discoloration include those of thrombophlebitis, allergic rashes, discoloring the skin of patients, hand foot syndromes, drug extravasations associated with the administration of the drug intravenously and drug induced nail changes. Diarrhea and constipation is observed as an adverse drug reaction in 6 percent of the adverse drug reactions. Nephrotoxicity is observed in 11 patients in the present study. Chemotherapeutic agents are known to cause both direct and indirect nephrotoxicity. Hepatotoxicity is observed in the 4 patients in our study accounting to 1 perecnt of the total adverse drug reactions. Anaphylaxis is observed in 4 patients in the present study. Death as an adverse event in the present study has been noticed in 2 patients accounting to less than 1 percent of all the adverse drug reactions documented [fig.10,table.6].

Assessment of preventability of the adverse drug reaction was done based on modified schumock and thornton scale[51]. Most of the adverse drug reactions belonged to the category "not preventable" However the more common reactions like nausea and vomiting belonged to the category of "preventable" adverse drug reactions.

Following Modified Schumock-Thornton algorithm was used to assess the preventability of the adverse drug reactions in the present study.

Criteria for determining preventability of an adverse drug reaction (ADR)
Section A
Answering "yes" to one or more of the following implies that an
ADR is DEFINITELY preventable
1. Was there a history of allergy or previous reactions to the drug?
2. Was the drug involved inappropriate for the patient's clinical condition?
3. Was the dose, route, or frequency of administration inappropriate for the patient's age, weight, or disease state?
If answers are all negative to the above, then proceed to Section B
Section B
Answering "yes" to one or more of the following implies that an
ADR is PROBABLY preventable
1. Was required therapeutic drug monitoring or other necessary laboratory tests not performed?
2. Was a documented drug interaction involved in the ADR?
3. Was poor compliance involved in the ADR?
4. Was a preventative measure not administered to the patient?

5. If a preventative measure was administered, was it inadequate and/or inappropriate? Answer 'NO' if this question is nonapplicable
If answers are all negative to the above, then proceed to Section C.
Section C
The ADR is NOT preventable

Over half (76%) of ADRs were classified as not preventable, 22% probably preventable and 2% of adverse drug reactions were definitely preventable according to the above mentioned scale. Most of the ADRs, assessed in commonly seen adverse drug reactions like nausea and vomiting were not preventable, but the study revealed that less than 40% of them were probably preventable and very few of them were definitely preventable. In the case of neutropenia about 25% of cases were found to be probably preventable and rest were not preventable. In the patients suffering from diarrhea or constipation, it was found out that 21% were probably preventable , the rest were not preventable (79%) which involved most of the patients who were prescribed oral capecitabine and oral lapatinib. Most of the patients suffering from neurotoxicity- which involved loss of sleep pattern, anorexia, depression, apprehension, anxiety and neuropathies were found out to be not preventable adverse drug reactions. Only 20% of the cases suffering neurotoxicity were found out to be probably preventable reactions. Nephrotoxicity was definitely preventable in 2 cases of the patients in whom we observed the reaction. In most of the patients nephrotoxicity was observed to be not preventable. Rest of the patients in whom we observed adverse drug reactions were those of alopecia, hepatotoxicity, skin discolouration, anaphylaxis and death as an adverse event were not preventable.

Some of the adverse drug reactions noticed in the study are : hand-foot syndrome due to capecitabine, oral mucosal lesions due to FEC regimen, localized allergic reaction due to docetaxel and bleomycin induced skin changes.

Fig. 11 - Image of hand in a patient suffering from hand-foot syndrome (HFS)

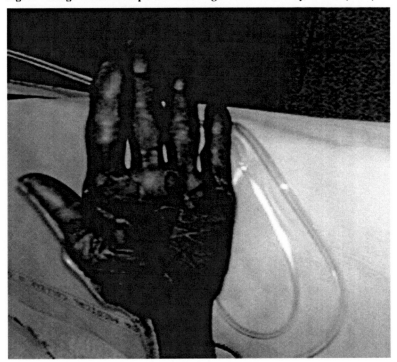

Fig. 12 - Image showing feet of patient suffering from hand – foot syndrome.

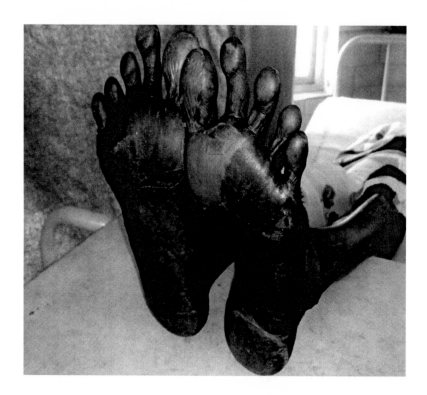

The grade-4 pattern of HFS with ulceration and desquamation over the soles.. The patient was prescribed vitamin biotin tablets and a healthy diet.

Fig. 13- Image of a patient showing the oral mucosal blackish discoloration due to FEC regimen for breast cancer.

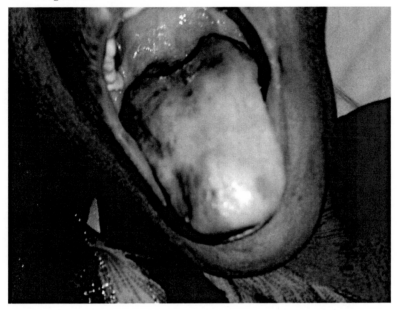

Fig. 14- Image of a patient showing localized allergic reaction due to i.v. docetaxel

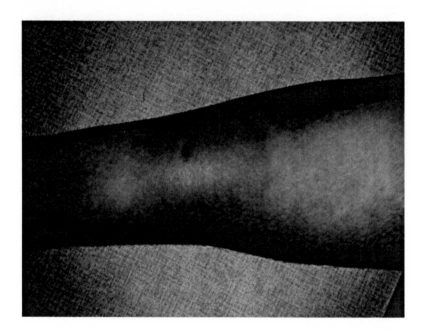

Fig. 15- Image of a patient showing the blackish discoloration over the lower back of a patient receiving bleomycin for testicular cancer.

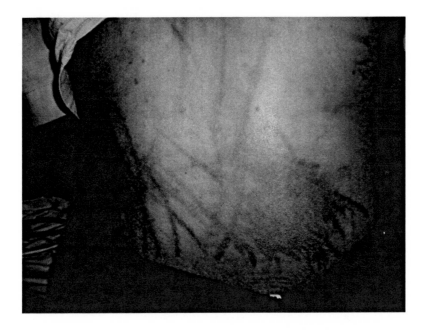

The patient had similar discoloration over the face, abdomen and limbs.

DISCUSSION

The main regimens used in our study are the FEC regimen[47,49] (5-fluorouracil, epirubicin and cyclophosphamide) for the breast cancer and cyclophosphamide/cisplatin and carboplatin/paclitaxel regimen for the ovarian cancer[49,50]. The general trend of adverse drug effects reported in the literature has already been mentioned. The naranjo algorithm scale for assessing adverse drug reactions was used to assess the severity of the reaction. Among the 202 patients, the percentage of females was 65% (131) and males was 35% (71), total number of adverse drug reactions were 898[master chart] as observed by bed to bed examination by residents with the help of lab diagnosis. Almost 53 percent of the adverse drug reactions according to naranjo algorithm were categorized as "probable" with score ranging from 5-8 and 47 percent were categorized as "possible" with score ranging from 1-4. Most of the adverse drug reactions were assumed to be moderately severe in variety according to the Hartwig scale.

This study has revealed an increase in the prevalence of patients suffering from breast cancer in the region, the cause of which is probably attributed to the increased use of oral contraceptives and alcohol consumption in the region. The western type of life style and type A personality bringing in early obesity in women is a likely cause of breast cancer. Awareness of the general population to the health related queries is also a cause for which women reach into the hospital and prove their presence in the hospital records[52]. Lesser use of the alkylating agents in the present study is in contrast to the study conducted in Bangladesh in the year 2009 and another study conducted in 1993 by Blacker. et.al, where alkylating agents were much more in common use, where as the present study agrees with the rule that women (females) suffer more from the anticancer therapy adverse drug effects than males [53]. The lesser use of the alkylating agents has been attributed to the intrinsic or acquired resistance to alkylating agents [54] which limit the therapeutic effects of the drugs. Because alkylating agents have narrow therapeutic index, the emergence of resistance can have significant impact upon the clinical success of the drugs[55]. These include alterations in drug uptake or drug efflux from the cell [transporter defects, P-glycoprotein (Mdr) overexpression], changes in drug-metabolizing enzymes [e.g., aldehyde dehydrogenase (cyclophosphamide), folylpolyglutamate synthetase (methotrexate), metallothionein (cisplatin)], and changes in target enzymes [dihydrofolate reducÃase (methotrexate), topoisomerase II (etoposide, teniposide), and enzymes of DNA repair [O6-methylguanine alkyltransferase]. Acquired resistance to chemotherapeutic drugs typically involves several independent mechanisms (multifactorial resistance) and can lead to cross-resistance to structurally unrelated drugs that exhibit distinct mechanisms of action. Recent studies have indicated that GSTs3 may play an important role in the resistance of cells and organisms not only to electrophilic herbicides, insecticides, and carcinogens but also to anticancer drugs as well. Nevertheless the relative success of alkylating agents in gaining therapeutic responses to diseases that are hard to treat continues to serve as an impetus to use alkylating moieties as a means to kill the cells. The increased use of natural products and anticancer antibiotics can be justified by the fact that there is rise in resistance to the alkylating agents as well as the sustained efforts of the oncologists for the search of newer products causing lesser adverse drug reactions.

The reasons for the increased incidence of ADRs in female patients may be due to the chemotherapeutic drugs displaying a wide inter individual variability in pharmacokinetics, which results in unpredictable toxicity in patients. Any factors that change the pharmacokinetics may easily cause toxicity due to their narrow therapeutic windows. Sex is one of the factors that contributes to the inter individual differences in pharmacokinetics. Sex difference in pharmacokinetics has been reported for numerous drugs, possibly because sex is easily identified and pharmacokinetics parameters are measurable[56]. Pharmacogenomics studies have revealed that the hepatic enzymes show a variation in their activity in different sexes. A phramacological explaination for the increase in adverse drug reaction rates in females may be due to lower body size and weight in females with consequent changes in apparent volume of distribution[57].

The maximum percentage of patients experiencing adverse drug reactions occurred in the age group between 50 and 59 years which accounted to 31 percent of patients in the study. The maximum percentage of the number of adverse drug reactions out of the total observed reactions, as compared to the age groups of the

64

patients was seen in the sixth decade [fig.8].The percentage prevalence of patients increased gradually forming a peak at the age group of 50-59 and then had a decline. The cause of old aged patients experiencing more number of adverse drug reactions can be attributed to the general biological processes in old age and change in the body surface area in the old age. However, the incidence of cancers is more common in the old age[57]. Finding that the adverse drug reactions according to the age group revealed an increase in the number of adverse drug reactions with every decade of patients' age till the age of 6th decade in the present study and then the decline in the number of adverse drug reactions in the further age group is similar to the study done by Richard. et .al. in England in the year 1998 [57]. Among the various adverse drug reactions assessed in the study, hematological toxicity is the most common to be observed. Among all the adverse drug reactions 29 percent of them was normocytic normochromic anaemia [fig.10]. The main toxicity of most anticancer agents is hematological, it corresponds to a decrease in the production of rapidly dividing cells such as blood cell progenitors[58,59]. These cells supply both self renewal and multi-lineage differentiation, and their role is to maintain the turnover of hematopoietic cells or to reverse cytopenia. Differentiated proliferating cells of each lineage are also sensitive to chemotherapy and take part in the process of cytopenia. Since circulating blood cells are not proliferating, immediate peripheral blood cell death plays a minor role in the myelotoxic process[60]. The findings in the present study are similar to those done by Retain et. al. in 1990 and Parchment et. al. in 1998. But the study differs in the fact that the percentage of patients suffering from hematological toxicity has been noted to be reduced. The cause of such reduction may be purported to the prophylactic use of maturation factors. The study revealed that 10 percent of patients suffered from neutropenia. Myelosuppression was the most common dose-limiting toxicity, noted in the treatment of various cancer patients. Neutropenia makes patients highly susceptible to pathogens resulting in life threatening infections or even death. Most common anticancer drugs causing myelosuppression are docetaxel, platinum drugs[61], and cyclophosphamide. Often the cause of neutropenia is the anticancer agent moieties in the circulation causing destruction of the colony forming blasts. There are various genes involved in the effects of anticancer drugs leading to neutropenia. Examples include the UGT gluconyltransferase gene and DPD genes involved in the pathways which lead to neutropenic influences by the anticancer drugs viz; 5-fluorouracil and irinotecan[62]. Elderly patients are more susceptible to the

65

toxicity of anticancer drugs. Elderly patients undergoing chemotherapy are at greater risk of neutropenia than are the younger age groups due to age related changes in the neutrophils. Studies have suggested that neutrophils in elderly patients are less phagocytic and are dysfunctional intracellular killers. Other patient related factors include female gender, poor nutritional status and comorbid conditions such as, diabetes, COPD, heart disease, and renal dysfunction[63].

The next common adverse drug reaction observed in the study was nausea/vomiting which formed 24 percent of total adverse drug reactions. The statistics of the study does not resemble those studies done in Bangladesh in the year 2009 (52 percent) by Sneegdha Poddar et. al and Mallik. S et. al. study done in Nepal in the year 2006 (44 percent), probably due to increased use of prophylactic antiemetics in the present study. The sensation of nausea and vomiting can be elicited by physiological, psychological, and environmental stimuli, such as an adverse drug reaction, post-operative changes during recovery, autonomic dysfunction, gastrointestinal dysfunction, mental stress, pain, smell, taste, motion, traumatic experiences, exposure to toxins, and many other stimuli. The major factors, which determine the incidence and severity of nausea and vomiting in patients receiving chemotherapy, include the dose and type of chemotherapy given, treatment schedule, the use of combinations of chemotherapeutic agents, and individual patient characteristics. The mechanism associated with the nausea and vomiting is due to stimulation of chemoreceptor trigger zone (CTZ) situated in the area postrema located on the dorsal surface of the medulla oblongata at the caudal end of the fourth ventricle. This area is not protected by the blood-brain barrier, and thus, can be reached by emetogenic chemicals via the cerebrospinal fluid or the blood. The essential region that coordinates vomiting is located in the brain stem between the levels of the obex and the retrofacial nucleus (just caudal to the facial nucleus). Within this region, the nucleus of the solitary tract (NTS) receives convergent input from different sources that can trigger vomiting, including the vagus nerve, area postrema, and vestibular and limbic systems. In turn, the NTS emits projections to the ventrolateral medulla and dorsal motor nucleus of the vagus. Projections to the ventrolateral medulla may be important for mediating the respiratory motor components of vomiting and those to the dorsal motor nucleus of the vagus for its gastrointestinal components. The interaction between this central neurocircuitry and the chemotherapeutic agent appears to be mediated by the release of neurotransmitters. Chemotherapeutic agents prompt the release of various neurotransmitters and neuropeptides, which in turn activate the vomiting center separately or in combination. Although the exact neurotransmitters that are released in the CTZ and vomiting center are not clearly defined, there is strong evidence that dopamine plays a role in mediating vomiting via the dopamine (D2) receptors[64].

Most of the chemotherapeutic drugs have been found to cause release of large amounts of serotonin from enterochromaffin cells in the gut, serotonin acts on 5-HT3 receptors in the gut and brain stem and stimulate vagal affarents to initiate the vomiting reflex. $5-HT_3$-receptor antagonists along with a corticosteroid are proved to be the key treatment regimen against CINV[65].

Alopecia was observed in 13 percent of patients in our study. However, the number of patients suffering total baldness was not more. Baldness was observed more commonly with the patients undergoing treatment with FEC regimen. The causes of the same can be attributed to the effects of alkylating agens and other chemotherapeutics to negatively affect the hair bulb growth and heterogeneity of hair progenitor sheath cells[66]. Alopecia is an unpreventable adverse drug reaction. Hair regrowth can be seen in most of the cases after the cessation of chemotherapy[67].

Neurotoxicity was observed in 6 percent of the adverse drug reactions in the study. The various features representing neurotoxicity associated with chemotherapy include nausea/vomiting, peripheral neuropathies, abdominal neuropathies, Loss of vibration sense, paraesthesia, ataxia and ototoxicity. The platinum drugs seem to affect the axons, myelin sheath, neuronal cell body, and the glial structures of the neurons. At the cellular level, the chemotherapy interferes with DNA replication and metabolic function of the neurons. Platinum-based agents have the propensity to enter the dorsal root ganglia and peripheral nerves as opposed to the brain, as these drugs have poor penetration through the blood-brain barrier. Levels of platinum have been shown to be significantly higher in the dorsal root ganglia than in the brain and spinal cord, which are protected by that barrier[68].

Skin discolouration - is observed in 6 percent of the patients with various adverse drug reactions in the present study. Various causes associated with skin discolouration include those of thrombophlebitis, allergic rashes discolouring the skin of patients, hand foot syndromes and drug extravasation associated with the administration of the drug intravenously, drug induced nail changes. Dose related acryl erythema is another type of dermatological complication specific to anticancer drugs use (Branzan et al., 2005)[69]. Chemotherapy induced mucocutaneous complications are common and in some cases more serious ones eg. erythema multiforme, but the cessation of causative agent is not necessary[69]. Pigmentation due to bleomycin in urology wards can be another cause of discolouration of skin.

Diarrhea and constipation is observed as an adverse drug reaction in 6 percent of the adverse drug reactions. The cuases of diarrhoea in the cancer chemotherapy patients is most commonly due to 5-fluorouracil, capecitabine, irinotecan[70] and alkylating agents. The absolute percentage of patients that have diarrhoea or constipation as a result of their treatment has yet to be fully defined, although general estimates place 10% of patients with advanced cancer as being afflicted in studies conducted in European countries[71]. Importantly, chemotherapy treatment also changes the composition of the native microflora within the intestine, although this has yet to be fully characterised. Normally, the microflora is involved in a number of gut functions, including but not limited to protection, metabolism of bilirubin, intestinal mucins, pancreatic enzymes, fatty acids, bile acids, cholesterol and steroid hormones. Other roles of gastrointestinal bacteria include nutrient processing, regulation of intestinal angiogenesis and immune functions. An alteration in the balance of microflora can result in a harmful environment existing within the intestine. The role of intestinal microflora in diarrhea has been highlighted recently, through investigations into the chemotherapeutic agent, irinotecan (CPT11), which causes severe diarrhea in the clinic[72]. Diarrhea and constipation are thought to be caused by the alteration in absorptive functions of cells, goblet cells and mucin distribution and composition and bacterial interactions with these cells and metabolites of the anticancer drugs themselves[73].Cytotoxic chemotherapy can cause functional and structural changes to the GIT. Common gastrointestinal symptoms following chemotherapy include heartburn, abdominal pain, diarrhoea (and constipation), bloating and nausea. These symptoms arise as the result of the damage caused by chemotherapy agents. Abdominal pain is caused by the extensive damage occurring in the small intestine. Diarrhoea and constipation are thought to be caused by the alteration in absorptive functions of cells, goblet cell and mucin distribution and composition, and bacterial interactions with these cells and metabolites of the drugs themselves. Cytotoxic drugs are known to act by inducing apoptosis in cancer , apoptosis is also induced in the GIT[71].

Nephrotoxicity is observed in 11 patients in the present study Chemotherapeutic agents are known to cause both direct and indirect nephrotoxicity. Agents used in the treatment of malignancy frequently cause acute but reversible toxicity to normal host proliferative tissues. Although the greatest toxicity is frequently in the bone marrow, skin, and gastrointestinal tissues, some agents are associated with renal toxicity. Indirect effects are primarily a consequence of tumor cell lysis and the resultant rapid release of large volumes of intracellular ions and metabolites. Direct renal toxicity has been described for multiple agents used for cancer chemotherapy. The agents most frequently associated with direct renal toxicity used in the treatment of malignancies include cisplatin, mitomycin-C, cyclophosphamide, and methotrexate. The effect of chemotherapy on the function of bladder, ureters and kidneys[74].

Nephrotoxicity is prevented by prechemotherapy hydration by fluids. Thus the present study has revealed only 2 percent of the total adverse drug reactions as nephrotoxicity.

Hepatotoxicity is observed in 4 patients in the present study accounting to 1 perecnt of the total adverse drug reactions. Almost all the alkylating agents do cause hepatotoxicity which can be observed in the lab reports of the patients by examining the hepatic enzymes levels by investigating hepatic liver function tests[75].

Anaphylaxis is observed in 4 patients in the present study. Hypersensitivity and anaphylaxis is a common occurrence with monoclonal antibody administration, alkylating agents, antibiotics and antimetabolites. Antihistamines and corticosteroids are used in the prevention of hypersensitivity reactions[16].In the present study, it has been noted that hypersensitivity with FEC regimen lead to the loss of life in one of the patients. Anaphylaxis accounted to 1 percent of all the adverse drug reactions.

Death as an adverse event in the present study has been noticed in 2 patients accounting to less than 1 percent among all the adverse drug reactions documented.

Adverse drug reactions (ADRs), including interactions, in older people are a common cause of admission to hospital, and are an important cause of morbidity and death[76]. The causes of death observed in the present study are anaphylaxis due to FEC regimen and neutropenic sepsis leading to death.

Itching, inflammation, headache, swelling, pleural effusions, loss of sleep and menstrual irregularities are some of the other adverse drug reactions observed in the study. To compensate these ADRs different classes of drugs were found to be used like proton pump inhibitor, vitamin, antibiotic, antiemetic, H2-receptor blocker viz, ranitidine, antiseptics, disinfectants, corticosteroids, anti-anemic, blood transfusion, sedatives, opiod analgesic, antispasmodic, antidepressant and antidiarrhoeals.

Biophysical charecteristics: the observation in the patients revealed that almost many of those patients treated on 5-flurouracil and capecitabine suffered gradual decline in the weight and thinning of the extremities.

Preventable adverse drug reaction was defined according to Schumock and Thornton (1992) as ADR which was preventable or avoidable. This criteria comprises of seven questions. The assessment is performed by answering "yes" or "no" to these questions based on the information of each adverse drug event.

1. Was the drug involved in the ADR not considered appropriate for the patient's clinical condition?
2. Was the dose, route, and frequency of administration not appropriate for the patient's age, weight and disease state?
3. Was required therapeutic drug monitoring or other necessary laboratory test not performed?
4. Was there a history of allergy or previous reactions to the drug?
5. Was a drug interaction involved in the reaction?
6. Was a toxic serum drug level documented?
7. Was poor compliance involved in the reaction?
The algorithm was expanded to include dispensing errors (errors at the dispensing stage in the pharmacy) and administration errors (errors when administering medication to the patient either by caretakers or by the patient, eg. nonadherence to

the medication regimen. Most of the adverse drug reactions belonged to the category "not preventable" However the more common reactions like nausea and vomiting belonged to the category of "definitely preventable".

Modified Schumock and thornton scale for preventability of adverse drug reaction assessment. Assessment of preventability of the adverse drug reaction was done based on modified schumock and thornton scale[51].

Criteria for determining preventability of an adverse drug reaction (ADR)
Section A
Answering "yes" to one or more of the following implies that an
ADR is DEFINITELY preventable
1. Was there a history of allergy or previous reactions to the drug?
2. Was the drug involved inappropriate for the patient's clinical condition?
3. Was the dose, route, or frequency of administration inappropriate for the patient's age, weight, or disease state?
If answers are all negative to the above, then proceed to Section B
Section B
Answering "yes" to one or more of the following implies that an
ADR is PROBABLY preventable
1. Was required therapeutic drug monitoring or other necessary laboratory tests not performed?
2. Was a documented drug interaction involved in the ADR?
3. Was poor compliance involved in the ADR?
4. Was a preventative measure not administered to the patient?
5. If a preventative measure was administered, was it inadequate and/or inappropriate? Answer 'NO' if this question is nonapplicable
If answers are all negative to the above, then proceed to Section C.
Section C
The ADR is NOT preventable

Over half (76%) of ADRs were classified as not preventable, 22% probably preventable and 2% definitely preventable according to the above mentioned scale. Most of the ADRs, assessed in commonly seen adverse drug reactions like nausea and vomiting were not preventable, but the study revealed that less than 40% of them were probably preventable and very few of them were definitely preventable. In the case of neutropenia about 25% of cases were found to be probably preventable and rest of them were not preventable. In the patients suffering from diarrhea or constipation, it was found out that 21% were probably preventable , the rest were not preventable (79%) which involved most of the patients who were prescribed oral capecitabine and oral lapatinib. Most of the patients suffering from neurotoxicity-which involved loss of sleep pattern , anorexia , depression, apprehension ,anxiety and neuropathies were found out to be not preventable adverse drug reactions. Only 20% of the cases suffering neurotoxicity were found out to be probably preventable reactions. Nephrotoxicity was definitely preventable in 2 cases of the patients in whom we observed the reaction. In most of the patients nephrotoxicity was observed to be not preventable. Rest of the patients in whom we observed adverse drug reactions were those of alopecia, hepatotoxicity, skin discolouration, anaphylaxis and death as an adverse event were not preventable. The finding of 2 percent adverse drug reactions, which are definitely preventable, is also revealed in the study by Phyllis M. Lau et. al. which was done on cancer patients in Australia in the year 2000[46].

Antiemetics like dexamethasone, ondensetron and ranitidine were the most common drugs used in the prevention of nausea/vomiting. GM-CSF was used to prevent neutropenia and sepsis associated with the same. Leucovorin injection,injection filgrastim and multivitamin tablets were used in the prevention of normocytic –normochromic anaemia and neutropenia. Mesna was used in the prevention of nephrotoxicity associated with ifosfamide and cyclophosphamide. Platinum drugs related nephrotoxicity was prevented by fluid overhydration.

CONCLUSIONS

ADRs are common in hospitalised oncology patients, predictable in many instances but definitely preventable in only a few. There are, however, many occasions where improved use of preventative measures has the potential to contribute to reducing the incidence and severity of ADRs. An understanding and appreciation of patients' perceptions of these events will help health-care professionals prioritise targeted interventions and prevention strategies. In summary, the number of patients observed in present one year study was 202. The percentage of adverse drug reactions was most commonly observed in the older age groups, viz. the age group between 50 and 59 years. Naranjo scale was the standard scale used for the causality assessment and the assessment of preventability of the adverse drug reaction was done based on modified Schumock and Thornton scale. The naranjo scale revealed that 53 percent of the adverse drug reactions according to naranjo algorithm were categorized as "probable" with score ranging from 5-8 and 47 percent were categorized as "possible" with score ranging from 1-4. Over half (76%) of ADRs were classified as not preventable, 22% probably preventable and 2% definitely preventable according to the above mentioned scale. Most of the ADRs, assessed in commonly seen adverse drug reactions like nausea and vomiting were not preventable, but the study revealed that less than 40% of them were probably preventable and very few of them were definitely preventable.

The most common adverse drug reactions observed in the study were those of the hematological toxicity followed by, gastrointestinal adverse drug effects, alopecia, neurotoxicity, skin toxicities and others. The study agreed to the law that women suffer more adverse drug reactions due to cancer chemotherapy than men do. We also deduced that the drugs used most commonly for preventing immediate adverse drug reactions were the antiemetics, followed by the corticosteroids.

The present study has also revealed the shift of use of the anticancer drugs from intravenous formulations to oral formulations e.g. use of i.v. 5-fluorouracil to oral doxifluridine (tab.carcidox). We thus conclude by the statement that the newer drug formulations for prevention of adverse drug reactions to cancer chemotherapy have been the main source for invention and discovery of new sources to decrease the morbidity associated with the anticancer drugs and their adverse effects.

A RARE CASE REPORT TO END THE STUDY

FEC –regimen causing bradycardia, fatal convulsions and death – a serious adverse drug reaction/event?

Abstract:- Breast cancer is one of the most common cause of death in the advanced countries , after heart disease, causing over 500,000 fatalities annually. The present role of FEC regimen has proved it to be the better initial treatment for carcinoma of breast. Anthracycline based chemotherapy is superior to non-anthracycline based regimens.Various adverse drug effects associated with the use of FEC regimen are – nausea, vomiting, alopecia , febrile neutropenia, fatigue , weight loss, diarrhea, myalgia , arthralgia, neuropathy , and premature ovarian failure. Some of the long term side effects include cardio toxicity and secondary cancers.Neurotoxicity with chemotherapy usually starts with CINV, bizarre dreams, cerebellar toxicity, convulsions and seizures are the other adverse drug reactions observed.

I report here a case of convulsions with seizures leading to death

Key words :-seizures , FEC regimen, neurotoxicity

Case report:

A 46 year old female , who was diagnosed with carcinoma of breast, stage 2,was advised inj.fluorouracil 500 mg/m2 infusion i.v. day 1 , inj.epirubicin 50 mg/m2 for 30 min infusion i. v. day 1, and inj.cyclophosphamide 500 mg/m2 infusion or bolus i.v.day 1 ,every 21 days for six cycles, after undergoing right sided modified radical mastectomy. No adverse drug reactions were observed in the patient other than nausea, vomiting, and anorexia after the first cycle of chemotherapy. The administration of second and the third cycle revealed that the patient suffered severe fall in the blood counts {as per the laboratory investigations} which was rectified by administering inj.GM-CSF 250 mcg/m2 iv once daily .The patient was admitted in the

74

ward for the fourth cycle in the morning and the process of infusion of the chemotherapeutic regimen was completed by 1800 hrs. None of the immediate untoward effects were observed other than nausea and vomiting which was controlled by administering inj. Ondensetron 2mg/ml i.v. At 2100 hrs the patient complained of blurred vision and changes in visual perception, abnormal light responses were observed. The patient was immediately shifted to the ICU and was found to be unconscious by the next half an hour. General physical examination revealed the blood pressure to be 60SBP/40DBP with bradycardia. Resuscitation efforts by the physician brought the blood pressure back to near normal i.e; 100SBP/70DBP. Dopamine was infused at the rate of 10μgm / kg/ min. The patient still remained unconscious, till 0200 hrs of the next day. Obvious convulsions and later GTCS were noted by the physician at 0230 hrs. As per the protocol inj.Lorazepam. i.v. 4mg was administered and repeated once after 10 min. Expected change in the patient's condition was not observed. Inj. Phenytoin was administered at the rate of 50 mg/min, yet the the status of the patient remained the same. Inj. Propofol. i.v.2mg/kg was administered and a slight improvement in the condition was noticed by the physician at 0300 hrs, but, the blood pressure was constantly falling and the patient could not be revived back to normal conditions despite of resuscitatory efforts by the physician. The general physical examination at the end revealed that the blood pressure was not recordable, and the heart beat could not be heard on auscultation. The pupillary reflex could not be elicited and was lost and ECG revealed a flatline lead and the patient was declared dead by 0400 hrs of the next day early morning hours.

Discussion- The mechanism of cardiotoxicity and neurotoxicity is not fully understood. It has been attributed by some authors to the conversion of alpha-fluorobeta-alanine, the major metabolite of FU, into fluoroacetate (FAC), which is known as a cardiotoxic and neurotoxic poison. Cardiotoxicity occurs during therapy with several cytotoxic drugs and may be the dose limiting factor in cancer treatment and hence tumour response. Cardiotoxicity includes a wide range of cardiac effects from small changes in blood pressure and arrhythmias to cardiomyopathy. The anthracyclines, such as doxorubicin and epirubicin, are potent cytotoxic drugs.The cause may be immunogenic.

BIBLIOGRAPHY

1) D C Classen, S L Pestotnik, R S Evans, J P Burke. Computerized surveillance of adverse drug events in hospital patients. Qual Saf Health Care 2005; 14:221–226.

2) Hitesh Patel, Derek Bell, Mariam Molokhia, Janakan Srishanmuganathan, Mitesh Patel, Josip car and Azeem Majid . Trends in hospital admissions for adverse drug reactions in England:analysis of national hospital episode statistics 1998–2005. BMC Clinical Pharmacology 2007; 10:1186-1472.

3) Lisa A. Ladewski, Steven M. Belknap, Jonathan R. Nebeker, Oliver Sartor, E. Allison Lyons, Timothy C. Kuzel, Martin S. Tallman, Dennis W. Raisch, Amy R. Auerbach, Glen T. Schumock, Hau C. Kwaan, and Charles L. Bennett . Dissemination of Information on Potentially Fatal Adverse Drug Reactions for Cancer Drugs From 2000 to 2002: First Results From the Research on Adverse Drug Events and Reports Project. Journal of Clinical Oncology. 2003; 21:3859-3866.

4) Jonathan R. Nebeker, Paul Barach , Matthew H. Samore, Clarifying Adverse Drug Events: A Clinician's Guide to Terminology, Documentation , and Reporting. Ann Intern Med. 2004;140:795-801

5) Scott A. Rivkees. Primum Non Nocere (First, Not to Harm) and Secundus, Opinio Vulnero (Second, Report the Harm). International Journal of Pediatric Endocrinology. 2009; 2009: 1155-1157

6) Kasper DL, Braunwald E, Fauci AS, Hauser SL, Longo DL, Jameson JL, Loscalzo J. Harrison's principles of internal medicine. 17th ed. New York: McGraw-Hill Medical Publishing Division; 2008

7) H.H.Hansen, D. F. Bajorin, H. B. Muss, G. Purkalne, D. Schrijvers & R. Stahel. Recommendations for a Global Core Curriculum in Medical Oncology. Annals of Oncology 2004;15:1603-1612

8) George J. Annas. An American Civil Liberties Union Handbook.3rd edition. Southern Illinois : University Press; 2004.

9) Laurence L Brunton, John S Lazo, Keith L Parker. Goodman and Gillman's The Pharmacological Basis of Therapeutics 11th edition. New York: McGraw-Hill; 2006.

10) Rose J. Papac. Origins of cancer therapy. Yale journal of biology and medicine 2001; 74:391-398.

11) Bertram G Katzung, Susan B Masters,Anthony J Trevor. Basic and clinical Pharmacology 11th edition. Tata McGraw-Hill. New Delhi; 2007.

12) I. Dávila González, R. Salazar Saeza,E. Moreno Rodilla,E. Laffond Ygesy, F. Lorente Toledano. Hypersensitivity reactions to chemotherapy drugs. Alergol Inmunol Clin. 2000;15:161-181.

13) Heinz-josef lenz. Management and Preparedness for Infusion and Hypersensitivity Reactions. The Oncologist. 2007;12:601–609.

14) Judy Hetherington, Caryn Andrews, Yaroslav Vaynshteyn and Rhonda Fishel. Managing follicular rash related to chemotherapy and monoclonal antibodies. Community Oncology.2007; 4:157-162.

15) Rudolph M. Navari. Overview of the updated antiemetic guidelines for chemotherapy-induced nausea and vomiting. Community Oncology. 2007;4:3-11

16) Hesketh PJ, Kris MG, Grunberg SM, et al. Proposal for classifying the acute emetogenicity of cancer chemotherapy. J Clincal Oncology. 1997; 15: 103–109.

17) Sydney M. Dy, Karl A. Lorenz, Arash Naeim, Homayoon Sanati, Anne Walling, and Steven M. Asch. Evidence-Based Recommendations for Cancer Fatigue, Anorexia, Depression, and Dyspnea. Journal of Clinical Oncology .2008;26:23-33.

18) Vainio A, Auvinen A. Prevalence of symptoms among patients with advanced cancer: An international collaborative study- Symptom Prevalence Group. J Pain Symptom Management. 1996; 12:3-10.

19) Lazzaro Repetto. Greater Risks of Chemotherapy Toxicity in Elderly Patients With Cancer. The Journal of Supportive Oncology . 2003;1:18–24

20) Lena E. Friberg, Anja Henningsson, Hugo Maas, Laurent Nguyen, and Mats O. Karlsson. Model of Chemotherapy-Induced Myelosuppression With Parameter Consistency Across Drugs.J Clin Oncol. 2002;20:4713–4721.

21) Giulia Fadda, Guglielmo Campus and PierFranca Lugliè. Risk factors for oral mucositis in paediatric oncology patients receiving alkylant chemotherapy. *BMC Oral Health* 2006; 6:13-18

22) M del Mar Sabater Recolons, José López López, M Eugenia Rodríguez de Rivera Campillo , Eduardo Chimenos Küstner , José María Conde Vidal ; Buccodental health and oral mucositis. Clinical study in patients with hematological diseases; Med Oral Patol Oral Cir Bucal 2006;11:E497-502.

23) Wilkes JD. Prevention and treatment of oral mucositis following cancer chemotherapy. Semin Oncol 1998;25:538-551.

24) Mustafa Baydar, MD; Mustafa Dikilitas, MD; Alper Sevinc, MD; and Ismet Aydogdu, MD Malatya and Gaziantep, Turkey; Prevention of Oral Mucositis Due to5-Fluorouracil Treatment with Oral Cryotherapy; JOURNAL OF THE NATIONAL MEDICAL ASSOCIATION. 2005;97:1161-1165

25) Perkins FM, Moxley RT, Papciak AS. Pain in multiple sclerosis and the muscular dystrophies. In: Block A, Kremer E, Fernandez E, editors. Handbook of pain syndromes. Mahwah, NJ: Erlbaum; 1999.

26) Verstappen CC, et al. Neurotoxic complications of chemotherapy in patients with cancer: Clinical signs and optimal management. Drugs.2003;63:1549-1563.

27) Johansson B, Mertens F, Heim S, Kristoffersson U, Mitelman F. Cytogeneticsofsecondary myelodysplasia (sMDS) and acute nonlymphocytic leukemia (sANLL). Eur J Hematol. 1991;47:17–27.

28) Geoffrey F Beadle, Alessandra Francesconi and Peter Baade, Acute myeloid leukemia after breast cancer: therapy related or host associated European journal of clinical & medical oncology 2010; 2:167-175.

29) Le Beau MM, Albain KS, Larson RA. Clinical and cytogenetic correlations in 63 patients with therapy-related myelodysplastic syndromes and acute nonlymphocytic leukemia: further evidence for characteristic abnormalities of chromosomes no 5 and 7. J Clin Oncol.1986; 4: 325–345.

30) CINDY L. SCHWARTZ, Long-Term Survivors of Childhood Cancer: The Late Effects of Therapy; The Oncologist 1999;4:45-54.

31) Mehmet Ali Erkurt, Ismet Aydogdu, Irfan Kuku, Emin Kaya and Onur Ozhan; Anticancer Drug Induced Glomerular Dysfunction; World Journal of Medical Sciences 2008;3 : 5-9.

32) Jing Zhang, Quan Tian and Shu-Feng Zhou; Clinical Pharmacology of Cyclophosphamide and Ifosfamide; Current Drug Therapy. 2006; 1: 55-84.

33) C. Bokemeyer, H.-J. Schmoll, E. Ludwig, A. Harstrick, T. Dunn & J. Casper; The antitumour activity of ifosfamide on heterotransplanted testicular cancer cell lines remains unaltered by the uroprotector mesna. Br. J. Cancer. 1994; 69:863-867

34) M.I. Gharib, A.K. Burnett. Chemotherapy-induced cardiotoxicity: current practice and prospects of prophylaxis; European Journal of Heart Failure. 2002;4: 235-242

35) Adriana Albini , Giuseppina Pennesi , Francesco Donatelli , Rosaria Cammarota, Silvio De Flora , Douglas M. Noonan; Cardiotoxicity of Anticancer Drugs: The Need for Cardio-Oncology and Cardio-Oncological Prevention.2010;102:440.

36) Peter Nygren . What is cancer chemotherapy? Acta Oncologica. 2001;40: 166–174.

37) M Eileen Dolan, R Stephanie Huang; Approaches to the discovery of pharmacogenomic markers in oncology: 2000–2010–2020 *Pharmacogenomics* .2010; 11: 471–474

38) S Marsh and HL McLeod. Cancer pharmacogenetics .British Journal of Cancer. 2004 ;90: 8 –11.

39) Martin J. Doherty. Algorithms for assessing the probability of an Adverse Drug Reaction. Respiratory Medicine CME. 2009;2: 63–67

40) WHO-UMC.The use of the WHO-UMC system for standardised case causality assessment.28 JULY 2005. Available from URL http://www.who-umc.org/pdfs/Causality.pdf .

41) *Andreea Farcas, Marius Bojita.* Adverse Drug Reactions in Clinical Practice: Causality Assessment of a Case of Drug-Induced Pancreatitis. J Gastrointestin Liver Dis. 2009;18: 353-358

42) Kishore pv, Subish palaian, Pradip ojha and Shankar pr pattern of adverse drug reactions experienced by tuberculosis patients in a tertiary care teaching hospital in western nepal; pak. j. pharm. sci. 2008;21: 51-56.

43) *Anne J. Leendertse, Antoine C. G. Egberts, Lennart J. Stoker,Patricia M. van den Bemt,* Frequency of and Risk Factors for Preventable Medication-Related Hospital Admissions in the Netherlands; (REPRINTED) ARCH INTERN MED.2008;168: 1890-1896.

44) Kannika Thiankhanithikun and Sayam Kaewvichit. Determination of Incidence and Characteristics of Preventable Adverse Drug Reactions: A Study in Phrae Hospital.CMU.J.Nat.Sci. 2009;8:55-62

45) Binayak Chandra Dwari, Surichhya Bajracharya, Pranaya Mishra, Subish Palaian, Smitha Prabhu, Mukhyaprana Prabhu. Morbilliform rashes due to erythromycin in a patient with herpes zoster infection. Journal of Pakistan Association of Dermatologists 2007; 17: 125-129.

46) Phyllis M. Lau, Kay Stewart, Michael Dooley. The ten most common adverse drug reactions (ADRs) in oncology patients:do they matter to you?. Support Care Cancer .2004;12:626–663

47) Monica Fornier and Larry Norton; Dose-dense adjuvant chemotherapy for primary breast cancer; Breast Cancer Res. 2005; 7:64-69.

48) Pierre Fumoleau, Jacques Bonneterre, Elisabeth Luporsi; Adjuvant Chemotherapy for Node-Positive Breast Cancer Patients: Which is the Reference Today? Journal of Clinical Oncology. 2003;21: 1190-1192.

49) *Martine J. et.al* .Randomized Intergroup Trial of Cisplatin–Paclitaxel Versus Cisplatin–Cyclophosphamide in Women With Advanced Epithelial Ovarian Cancer: Three-Year Results; Journal of the National Cancer Institute. 2000;92:699-709.

50) P. Zola & A. Ferrero; Is carboplatin–paclitaxel combination the standard treatment of elderly ovarian cancer patients? Annals of Oncology .2007;10:1483-1485

51) Waraporn Srisuwannarat. Role of pharmacist in the prevention of potentially preventable adverse drug reactions in general medicine wards at ramathibodhi hospital. Mahidol university. Fac Mahidol University. 2007.

52) Sinha.R, Anderson.D.E, Macdonald.S.S, Greenwald.P, Cancer risk and diet in India, Journal of Post Graduate Medicine .2003;49:222-228

53) Sneegdha Poddar, Razia Sultana, Rebeka Sultana, Maruf Mohammad Akbor,Mohammad Abul Kalam Azad and Abul Hasnat; Pattern of Adverse Drug Reactions Due to Cancer Chemotherapy in Tertiary Care Teaching Hospital in Bangladesh; Dhaka Univ. J. Pharm. Sci. 2009;8:11-16.

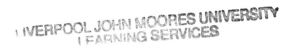

54) By Vincent T. DeVita, Theodore S. Lawrence, Steven A. Rosenberg, Robert A. Weinberg, Ronald A.; DeVita, Hellman, and Rosenberg's cancer: principles & practice of oncology. Newyork; Lippincott Williams.2007.

55) David j Waxman. Glutathione 5-Transferases: Role in Alkylating Agent Resistance and Possible Target for Modulation Chemotherapy-A Review; Cancer research. 1990; 50:6449-6454.

56) Jeffrey Wang and Ying Huang; Pharmacogenomics of Sex Difference in Chemotherapeutic Toxicity; Current Drug Discovery Technologies. 2007;4: 59-68.

57) Richard M Martin et. Al.; age and sex distribution of suspected adverse drug reactions to newly marketed drugs in general practice in England; analysis of 48 cohort studies. British journal of clinical Pharmacology; 1998;46: 505-511.

58) Ratain MJ, Schilsky RL, Conley BA, Egorin MJ. Pharmacodynamics in cancer therapy. J Clin Oncol. 1990;8:1739–1753.

59) Parchment RE, Gordon M, Grieshaber CK, Sessa C,Volpe D, Ghielmini M. Predicting hematological toxicity (myelosuppression) of cytotoxic drug therapy from in vitro tests. Ann Oncol. 1998;9:357–364.

60) Diane Testart-Paillet, Pascal Girard Benoit You Gilles Freyer, Christian Pobel, Brigitte Tranchand, Contribution of modelling chemotherapy-induced hematological toxicity for clinical practice; Critical Reviews in Oncology/ Hematology .2007;63: 1–11.

61) Charlotte Kloft, JohanWallin, Anja Henningsson, Etienne Chatelut, and Mats O.Karlsson; Population Pharmacokinetic-Pharmacodynamic Model for Neutropenia with Patient Subgroup Identification: Comparison across Anticancer Drugs; Clin Cancer Res 2006;12: 5481-5491.

62) Mouldy Sioud; Methods in molecular biology.Ne jersey:Humana Press;2007.

63) Lee s Schwartzberg. Neutropenia ; Etiology and pathogenesis; Clinical corner stone .2006;8: 5 –11.

64) Abhay r. Shelke, Karen m. Mustian and Gary r. Morrow; the pathophysiology of treatment-related nausea and vomiting in cancer patients : current models; indian j physiol pharmacol. 2004; 48 : 256–268.

81

65) Sayantani Ghosh, Saugat Dey; Comparing Different Antiemetic Regimens for Chemotherapy Induced Nausea and Vomiting; *International Journal of Collaborative Research on Internal Medicine & Public Health.* 2010;2: 142-156.

66) Yasuyuki Amoh1,2,3, Lingna Li1, Kensei Katsuoka2 and Robert M. Hoffman1,3; Chemotherapy Targets the Hair-Follicle Vascular Network but Not the Stem Cells ; Journal of Investigative Dermatology. 2007;127:11–15.

67) Milly E de Jonge, Ron AA Mathôt, Otilia Dalesio, Alwin DR Huitema, Sjoerd Rodenhuis, Jos H Beijnen; Relationship between irreversible alopecia and exposure to cyclophosphamide, thiotepa and carboplatin (CTC) in high-dose chemotherapy; *Bone Marrow Transplant. 2002; 30: 593-597.*

68) Sarah R. McWhinney, Richard M. Goldberg,and Howard L. McLeod;Platinum neurotoxicity pharmacogenetics; Mol Cancer Ther. 2009;8:10–16.

69) Noor kamil, Saba kamil, Shahida p. Ahmed, Rizwan Ashraf,Mohammad Khurram and Muhammad Obaid Ali; toxic effects of multiple anticancer drugs on skin; pak. j. pharm. sci.2010;23:7-14

70) Renée J. Goldberg Arnold, Nashat Gabrail, Monika Raut, Renée Kim, Jennifer C. Y. Sung, MS, and Yonglong Zhou; Clinical Implications of Chemotherapy-induced Diarrhea in Patients With Cancer; J Support Oncol. 2005;3:227–232.

71) Andrea M. Stringer, Rachel J. Gibson, Joanne M. Bowen and Dorothy M.K. Keefe; Chemotherapy-Induced Modifications to Gastrointestinal Microflora: Evidence and Implications of Change. *Current Drug Metabolism.*2009; *10:* 79-83.

72) Joanne M. Bowen1, Andrea M. Stringer, Rachel J. Gibson Ann S.J. Yeoh ,Sarah Hannam; Dorothy M.K. KeefeVSL#3 Probiotic Treatment Reduces Chemotherapy-Induced diarrhea and weight loss; Cancer Biology & Therapy .2007 ;6:61-66.

73) Mitchell EP, Schein PS. Gastrointestinal Toxicity of Chemotherapeutic Agents. In: Derry MC, Yabro JW, eds. Toxicity of Chemotherapy. New York: Grune & Stratton Inc; 1984:269–285.

74) Michael e. Carley; The effect of chemotherapy on the function of bladder,ureters and kidneys; CME Journal of Gynecologic Oncology. 2002; 7:100 –102.

75) Paul d. King,Michael c. Perry, Hepatotoxicity of Chemotherapy; The Oncologist. 2001;6:162-176.

76) P. A. Routledge, M. S. O'Mahony1 & K. W. Woodhouse; Adverse drug reactions in elderly patients; British Journal of Clinical Pharmacology; Br J Clin Pharmacol. 57:2 121–126.

ABBREVIATIONS

1) ADR-adverse drug reaction
2) ADR's- adverse drug reactions
3) FDA- food and drug administration
4) VOD- venoocclusive disease
5) CINV-Chemotherapy induced nausea and vomiting
6) FEC-5 Fluorouracil,epirubicin,cyclophosphamide
7) CP-Carboplatin/Paclitaxel
8) CC-Cisplatin,Cyclophosphamide
9) Mdr- Multidrug resistant
10) GM-CSF- granulocyte-monocyte colony stimulating factor
11) i- injection
12) tab.-tablet
13) Ont.-ointment
14) ADE-adverse drug event
15) pADRs-preventable adverse drug reactions
16) Cll- chronic lymphocytic leukaemia
17) Nna- normocytic normochromic anemia
18) CML-chronic myeloid leukemia
19) ALL- acute lymphocytic leukaemia
20) DNA-deoxy ribose nucleic acid
21) AML-acute myeloid leukaemiakin's
22) NHL-non-hodgkin's lymphoma
23) SIADH-Syndrome of Inappropriate Secretion of Antidiuretic Hormone
24) ILD-interstitial lung disease

Sr.No.	Name	age	sex	diagnosis	Rx given
1	kashinath naik	55	m	esophageal ca	i5fu,icisplatin
2	prashant	77	m	glioma	temozolomide tab
3	maria gomes	55	f	ca breast	cyclophosphamide,epirubicin,5fu
4	uttara manerikar	54	f	ca breast	deca,pantoprazole,ondem,idocetaxel,l doxorubicin
5	kajesab dandir	14	f	osteosarcoma	idoxirubicin,icisplatin,imethotrxate
6	santana a fernandes	38	f	ca of ovary	icarboplatin ,ipaclitaxel
7	parvatishivaprabhu	56	f	ca breast	idocetaxel,icyclophosphamide,iepirubicin
8	uttamamanenkar	54	f	ca breast	idocetaxel,icyclophosphamide,iepirubicin
9	mallarikhamble	62	m	caofstomach	i5fu,ileucovorin
10	revati naik	50	f	ca of rectum	iirinotecan ,5fu,ileucovorin
11	urmila vinayak	44	f	ca of ovary	icarboplatin ,ipaclitaxel
12	lazarina felix fernandes	44	f	ca of ovary	ipaclitaxel,carboplatin
13	vasanti shirodkar	35	f	caof buccalmucosa	i5fu,icisplatin
14	pramod haldankar	42	m	ca supraglottis	icisplatin,i5fu
15	paulo d,souza	63	m	multiple myeloma	icyclophosphamide
16	anil palkar	36	m	non hodgkins disease	iadriamycin,ivinblastine,ibleomycin,icyclophosphamide
17	domingos mascarhenas	66	m	ca colon	i5fu
18	prakash chari	52	m	ca larynx	icisplatin,5fu
19	shobha hawnoor	36	f	ca esophagus	tab carcidox
20	manorama naik	55	f	ca breast	icyclophosphamide,iepirubicin,t carcidox
21	sujal satardekar	45	f	ca breast	iepirubicin,t.carcidox,icyclophosphamide
22	xareena fernandes	37	f	ca breast	icyclophosphamide,iepirubicin,t carcidox
23	govind gawade	55	m	ca sigmoid colon	i5fu,ileucovorin
24	santosh naik	45	m	ca of oral cavity	icisplatin,i5fu,ileucovorin
25	sumitra ramnath	39	f	ca breast	icyclophosphamide,iepirubicin,i5fu
26	prakash yogi	17	m	nasopharyngeal ca	icisplatin,5fu
27	laxmi kamble	65	f	multiple myeloma	icyclophosphamide
28	narayan ratwad	58	m	waldenstroms macroglobulinaemia	irituximab,icyclophosphamide
29	laxmi mogra	46	f	ca breast	idocetaxel,icyclophosphamide,i5fu,iepirubicin
30	shantabai pai	60	f	ca of rectum	i5fu
31	aparna lingoji	35	f	ca breast	icyclophosphamide,iepirubicin,i5fu(idocetaxel,icyclophosphamide)
32	bharati mohan mapsekar	80	f	ca breast	idocetaxel,tabcarcidox
33	sumitra narvekar	50	f	ca breast	icyclophosphamide,i5fu,iepirubicin
34	geeeta sawanth	55	f	cabreast	iFEC
35	amelia mendes	53	f	cabreast	icef,t.capecitabine,t.lapatinib,i.docetaxel
36	neeta mandrekar	50	f	cabreast	iFEC
37	indrayani shet	44	f	nhl	ichop
38	rihana	49	f	caovary serous cystadenoca	icarboplatin ,ipaclitaxel
39	tommy soares	55	m	capyriform fossa	icisplatin,i5fu
40	murtaza muzzaffar	45	m	caoral cavity	tab carcidox
41	shobha naik	42	f	ca of rectum	tab carcidox,idocetaxel
42	devata tamankar	55	f	glioma	tab.temozolamide
43	lavina costa	10	f	nhl	ichop
44	mirabai thawte	79	f	nhl	iCHOP,rituximomab
45	ashvini loltikar	60	f	cabreast	iFEC
46	vincentina fernandes	45	f	nhl	iCHOP
47	monabaishirodkar	58	f	ca ovary	icarboplatin ,ipaclitaxel
48	ramakant bandodkar	42	m	ca supraglottis	t.carcidox
49	avin velip	5.5	m	astrocytoma	icyclophosphamide,mesna,cisplatin,i,vincristine
50	shantabai gawas	58	f	ca breast	icyclophosphamide,adriamycin,t.carcidox
51	priya chodankar	40	f	cabreast	idocetaxel,t.carcidox
52	sujatasurajnaik	28	f	cabreast	iadriamycin,icyclophosphamide,t.carcidox

#	Name	Age	Sex	Diagnosis	Treatment
53	neeta mandrekar	50	f	cabreast	tab.capacitabine,tab.lapatinib,j.docetaxel
54	severina dsouza	63	f	cabreast	tab.capacitabine,tab.lapatinib,j.docetaxel
55	shamsuna suleman	48	f	cabreast	iFEC
56	angela falcao	65	f	cabreast	iFEC
57	sumitra pagi	39	f	cabreast	iFEC
58	gopiki khandeparkar	60	f	ca ovary	icyclophosphamide,icisplatin
59	concessao borges	62	f	ca ovary,stage3	ipacilitaxel,carboplatin
60	aryan nadaf	5	m	all	intrathecal mtx,idoxorubicin,jasparaginase,ivincristine
61	gavin	5	m	alll3	ivcr,l i-asparaginase,idaunorubicin,tabmtx
62	jasmine laurdes	55	f	ca colon	ioxaliplatin,tabcapecitabine
63	shailu naik	58	f	glioma	tabtemozolamide
64	matthew cordozo	69	m	castomach	idocetaxel,tabcarcidox
65	radha raut	56	f	ca breast	idocetaxel,tabcarcidox
66	geeta naik	43	f	cabreast	idocetaxel,t.carcidox
67	shilpatalkatkar	38	f	cabreast	iadriamycin,icyclophosphamide,t.carcidox
68	seetabai gadekar	60	f	cabreast	ioxaliplatin,i5fu,ileucovorin
69	heeradevi singh	70	f	cabreast	icyclophosphamide,tab.carcidox,iadriamycin
70	nutan sambhari	50	f	cabreast	icyclophosphamide,iepirubicin,5fu
71	kalpana gaunkar	52	f	cabreast	tcarcidox,iepirubicin,icyclophosphamide
72	gulfareen khatib	14	f	caovary serous cystadenoca	ietoposide,icisplatin,ibleomycin
73	concessica pereira	49	f	cabreast	icyclophosphamide,iepirubicin,t carcidox
74	shubhanginavelkar	38	f	cabreast	icyclophosphamide,iadriamycin,5fu
75	pradeep salelkar	30	m	cml	tab imatinib,i cytarabine
76	kamalakant harmalkar	70	f	ca rectum	ioxaliplatin,tabcarcidox
77	ranjitnaik	23	m	seminomatestis	icisplatin,ietoposide,ibleomycin
78	ashalaxmandhumaskar	62	f	caovary serous cystadenoca	icarboplatin ,ipaclitaxel
79	kovin mahale	20	m	pnet	ivincristine,jifosphamide,ietoposide,imesna
80	joshna more	27	f	retroperitoneal mass	ivincristine,icyclophosphamide,iepirubicin
81	adriana carvalho	65	f	ca ovary	icarboplatin ,ipaclitaxel
82	santosh goltekar	47	m	fibrosarcoma	iifosphamide,idoxorubicin
83	gurudas narvekar	62	f	ca rectum	ioxaliplatin,ileucovorin,i5fu,ibevacizumab
84	sunaina bhosle	28	f	ca ovary	icisplatin,ietoposide
85	netra naik	57	f	cabreast	icyclophosphamide,iadriamycin,tabcarcidox
86	padmaja patil	39	f	cabreast	iFEC
87	suman vast	65	f	caovary serous cystadenoca	iFEC
88	radhabai naik	65	f	cabreast	icyclophosphamide,icisplatin
89	sushmaprakash	58	f	cabreast	icyclophosphamide,iadriamycin,tabcarcidox
90	neelima chorlekar	25	f	caovary	icyclophosphamide,iepirubicin,i5fu
91	vimal naik	40	f	caovary	icyclophosphamide,icisplatin
92	pooja desai	36	f	ca cervix	icisplatin
93	ganpat narvekar	50	m	cacachexia	ifu
94	bhagirathi gawas	50	f	cabreast	icyclophosphamide,iepirubicin,5fu
95	noor bi khan	57	f	ca breast	icyclophosphamide,i5fu,iepirubicin
96	vimal joshilkar	45	f	ca breast	icyclophosphamide,iepirubicin,t carcidox
97	santana dias	50	f	cabreast	icyclophosphamide,iadriamycin,t.carcidox
98	anand gaonkar	25	m	ca rectum	ioxaliplatin,iBevacizumab,i5fu,ileucovorin
99	susheela kothwale	50	f	ca tongue	idocetaxel,i5fu,ileucovorin
100	mahadevi g naik	40	f	ca breast	icyclophosphamide,i5fu
101	flavian d'souza	67	m	all	iprednisolone,i6mp,ilasp,tmtx,ivcr
102	suman vaman naik	50	f	ca breast	icyclophosphamide,i5fu
103	maya velip	35	f	ca breast	iFEC
104	shubhangi desai	44	f	ca ovary	iadriamycin,icyclophosphamide,t.carcidox icyclophosphamide,icisplatin
105	kalpana desai	66	f	glioma	t.temozolomide

#	Name	Age	Sex	Diagnosis	Treatment
106	rosario gomes	54	m	nhl	icyclophosphamide,ivcr,idoxorubicin
107	vilas redkar	46	m	ca rectum	i5fu
108	devendra chopdekar	50	m	ca tongue	icisplatin,5fu,ileucovorin
109	dattaram mulgaonkar	62	m	oral ca	icisplatin,idocetaxel,t.carcidox
110	deirdre da costa	12	f	aml	idaunomycin,iara-c,t.6tg,t.prednisolone
111	sunita chari	55	f	aml	icytarabine,idaunorubicin,ifilgrastim,6tg,6mp
112	sebastiana andrade	45	f	ca breast	iFEC
113	rupesh koltekar	20	m	recurrent osteosarcoma	idoxirubicin,icisplatin
114	sushma gaonkar	28	f	gestational trophoblastic disease	ivcr,icyclophosphamide,idactinomycin,imtx,ietoposide
115	shubhangi gawli	38	f	ca breast	icyclophosphamide,iepirubicin,t.carcidox
116	sarita haldankar	57	f	cabreast	icyclophosphamide,iadriamycin,t.carcidox
117	ermelina d'souza	60	f	cabreast	icyclo,iepirubicin,t.carcidox
118	shubha agni	58	f	ca peritoneum	igemcitabine,icisplatin
119	maria fernandes	2	f	wilms tumor	ivcr,idactinomycin
120	lala sab	27	f	hodgkins disease	i ABVD
121	nandita	45	f	cabreast	icyclophosphamide,iepirubicin,t.carcidox
122	potu gawde	65	m	caesophagus	i5fu,icisplatin
123	fatimabi sayyad	65	f	cabreast	icyclophosphamide,iepirubicin,t.carcidox
124	laxmi kadam	36	f	castomach	i5fu,ileucovorin
125	numnath borkar	75	m	ca colon	i5fu,ileucovorin
126	bebi kolvekar	35	f	cabreast	icyclophosphamide,iepirubicin,i5flurouracil
127	shreya naik	32	f	cabreast	icyclophosphamide,iepirubicin,i5flurouracil
128	krishna walvekar	51	m	nhl	i5fu,ileucovorin
129	hari bhuskute	71	m	ca stomach	i5fu,ileucovorin
130	malti awarsekar	51	f	cabreast	icyclophosphamide,iepirubicin,ifu
131	pranali adpaikar	36	f	cabreast	icyclophosphamide,i5fu,iiepirubicin
132	anthony fernandes	54	m	ca colon	ioxaliplatin,tab.capecitabine
133	nandita naresh naik	45	f	cabreast	l docetaxel,ilapatinib,tcapecitabine
134	moimuddin shaikh	65	m	capharynx	icisplatin,i5fu
135	mehboob mulla	20	m	aml	i6mp,ietoposide,iasparaginase,idaunorubicin
136	pranata gawas	5	f	retinoblastoma	icarboplatin,ietoposide,ivincristine,cap.endoxan,icyclosporine
137	shevanti kobal	54	f	ca rectum	ioxaliplatin,t.carcidox
138	shiva madkaikar	60	m	ca lung	icisplatin,igemcitabine
139	victor gonsalves	73	m	ca lung	icisplatin,ietoposide
140	francis d'souza	60	m	ca lung	icisplatin,,l etoposide
141	rohini borkar	58	f	ca lung	icisplatin,l etoposide
142	jyotiba panne	54	m	calung	icisplatin,igemcitabine
143	brigita dias	58	f	calung	icisplatin,igemcitabine
144	anton rodrigues	53	m	calung	icarboplatin,itaxol
145	inas mascerhas	64	m	calung	icisplatin,l etoposide
146	baburao naik	65	m	calung	icisplatin,igemcitabine
147	narayan chari	71	m	calung	icisplatin,igemcitabine
148	raghuri naik	60	m	calung	icisplatin,igemcitabine
149	shankar shirodkar	56	m	calung	icisplatin,igemcitabine
150	datta naik	70	m	calung	icisplatin,ietoposide
151	babuli mulla	70	m	calung	icisplatin,J gemcitabine
152	arjun kholkar	60	m	calung	icisplatin,l etoposide
153	ramakant phadte	53	m	calung	icisplatin,ietoposide
154	arabella fernandes	75	f	cabreast	icyclophosphamide,iepirubicin,i5fu
155	vijayashekhar hori	49	f	cabreast	icyclophosphamide,iepirubicin,i5fu
156	vinanti solyekar	35	f	cabreast	icyclophosphamide ,iepirubicin,i5fu
157	many fernandes	76	f	cabreast	icyclophosphamide ,iepirubicin,i5fu
158	ashwini lotlikar	60	f	cabreast	icyclophosphamide,iepirubicin,i5fu

159	salvador simeos	62	m	ca colon	i5fu
160	shashikant naik	60	m	ca colon	icarboplatin ,idocitaxel
161	prabhavati mandrekar	52	f	ca cervix	icisplatin
162	nayana kasutikar	48	f	ca ovary	icarboplatin,ipacitaxel
163	gopika faldesai	52	f	ca ovary	icarboplatin ,i pacitaxel
164	jyotsna palyekar	56	f	ca breast	iFEC
165	sridhar goingudda	6	m	all	i6mp,imtx,ivcr,iprednisolone
166	harichandra palni	64	m	ca glottis	icisplatin,i5fu
167	ayesha be shaik	62	f	ca breast	iFEC
168	zamira soares	63	f	ca colon	ioxaliplatin,icetuximab,i5fu,ileucovorin
169	yeshwant desai	57	m	ca stomach	irinotecan and 5fu,ileucovorin
170	chandrakala rawool	45	f	anaplastic oligodendroglioma	t.temozolomide
171	prajot naik	8	m	all	ivcr,iasparaginase,imtx,idaunorubicin,iprednisolone
172	rupali	36	f	ca ovary	ipacitaxel,carboplatin
173	imamsab kojurnoor	28	m	testicular tumor	icisplatin,ietoposide,bleomycin
174	chandravati jalmi	70	f	ca larynx	icisplatin,i5fu
175	sumita tarkar	39	f	ca oralcavity	icisplatin,5fu,ileucovorin
176	rosario periera	55	m	ca hepatic flexure	i5fu,ileucovorin
177	vijdosav borges	65	m	nhl	irituximab,ivcr,idoxorubicin,icyclophosphamide,iprednisolone
178	cyrilo fernandes	50	m	ca stomach	i5fu,ileucovorin
179	mita devi	56	f	ca brain	ttemozolomide
180	cosma souza	36	m	ca brain	ttemozolomide
181	jayanti chari	46	f	ca breast	iFEC
182	tulsidas naik	40	m	ca rectum	ioxaliplatin,i5fu,ileucovorin
183	laxmi naik	61	f	ca supraglottis	l cisplatin,5fu
184	archana sawant	40	f	ca breast	icyclophosphamide,iepirubicin,t carcidox
185	sugrambi khatib	52	m	ca breast	icyclophosphamide,iepirubicin,t carcidox
186	bibi zeare	60	f	ca breast	iFEC
187	kashi gawde	48	f	ca ovary	ipacitaxel,carboplatin
188	chandra karole	55	f	ca cervix	icisplatin,i5fu
189	sarita angle	53	f	ca breast	icyclophosphamide,iadriamycin,t.carcidox
190	noorjahan agha	64	f	ca colon	i5fu,ileucovorin
191	maria fernandes	55	f	ca colon	i5fu,ileucovorin
192	subha agni	58	f	ca ovary	icisplatin,igemcitabine,icarboplatin ,I paclitaxel
193	nirmala phadte	52	f	ca oralcavity	icisplatin,icyclophosphamide
194	rekha podalkar	50	f	ca ovary	icisplatin,i5fu
195	saroja shirodkar	49	f	ca ovary	ipacitaxel,carboplatin
196	ulhas chari	42	m	ca oralcavity	ipacitaxel,icisplatin
197	mahadev gaonkar	50	m	ca glottis	icisplatin,i5fu
198	ashrat bi khan	56	f	ca glottis	icarboplatin,ipacitaxel
199	sarita chimalkar	48	f	ca ovary	icyclophosphamide,icisplatin
200	bala bhandari	36	m	ca supraglottis	icisplatin,i5fu,ileucovorin
201	parvati prabhu	45	f	ca breast	idocetaxel,iadriamycin,icyclophosphamide
202	sheela.m	17	f	ca ovary	icarboplatin,ipacitaxel

adr	number of reactions	hospital no.
neutropenia	1	80012420
nausea,vomiting	1	80045320
alopecia,constipation,thrombophlebitis	3	90002341
nna,angioedema,anaphylactic rash over the skin over hips,alopecia,mucosal ulcerations,eczematous rash at the injection site	6	34961
normocytic normochromic anaemia	1	900075469
nna,headache	1	900076732
nna,decreased platelet count,nausea,vomiting,abdpain,legs and hand pain,alopecia	7	900014367
folliculitis,gum inflammation,nausea vomiting	4	900019512
discolouration of upper left limb,nna	2	900014044
decreased neutrophil count,nna	2	800045830
nausea,vomiting,nna,guiddiness,alopecia,constipation	6	900076128
nna,neutropenia	2	900016722
vomiting,nna,thrombocytopenia,neutropenia,diarrhoea	5	900071971
nna	1	900072307
gross heamaturia,nephrotoxicity	2	900041134
nna	1	900042534
nna,nausea,vomiting	3	900029114
nna	1	900022251
nna,nausea,vomiting,loose motion	4	800035353
nna	1	900047917
nausea,vomiting,alopecia,nna	4	900035478
nna,nausea,vomiting,alopecia	4	724503
pain at injection site,nna	2	900023232
nausea, vomiting,nna	3	90003514
nna,vomiting,nausea,alopecia	4	900025871
nna,vomiting,nausea	3	900044944
nna	1	900058511
nna,neutropenia,fever	3	984528617
nna,alopecia,hand foot syndrome,headache,thrombophlebitis,nausea	6	900020105
nna,injection site pain,oral mucosal leisions	3	800047339
urticaria,anaphylaxis,nna,peripheral neuropathy,alopecia,nausea,vomiting	7	900082545
nna,nausea,vomiting,alopecia,neutropenic sepsis,death	5	900033597
nna,nausea,vomiting,diarrhoea,alopecia	5	900029040
nna,anorexia	2	59377
nna,vomiting,diarrhoea,nausea,anorexia,alopecia,blackening of tongue and hands	7	900066907
nna,loosemotions,blackening of hand and foot	3	9000854721
nna,nausea,neutropenia,alopecia	4	9000465272
nna,neutropenia,nausea,vomiting,diarrhoea,hepatotoxicity	5	900023461
alopecia,constipation,headache,vomiting,unilateral limb edema(rul)	4	9033388221
nausea,vomiting,diarrhoea,thrombophlebitis	5	90022134442
nna,nausea,vomiting,ivsitepain,alopecia	5	900026571
vomiting	1	900026783
nna,alopecia,thrombophlebitis	3	900023651
nna,nausea,vomiting,anaphylactic rash	4	900004542
nna	1	900094604
nna	1	80007865
nna,neutropenia,nausea,vomiting,anaphylaxis,cough,alopecia,heamaturia,pain at iv site,neuropathy,nephrotoxicity	10	800043757
nausea	1	900010727
nna,nausea,vomiting,alopecia,neutropenia,infections,alopecia,anorexia	8	800045932
nna,neutropenia,nausea,vomiting,alopecia	5	900055055
nna,anorexia,limbpain,alopecia	4	900042005
nna,anorexia,vomiting,nausea	4	900056741

Symptoms	Count	ID
nna,neutropenia,thrombocytopenia,hand and foot syndrome,,alopecia,diarrhoea	6	900085474
alopecia,neutropenia,nna,hand foot syndrome	4	900042437
nausea,vomiting,nna,anorexia,alopecia	5	9000062373
alopecia,vomiting,nausea,tremor,thrombophlebitis	5	900009082
nna,neutropenia,thrombocytopenia,alopecia,hepatotoxicity,anaphylaxix,peripheral neuropathy,,discolouration of nails,menses loss	8	900025871
nna,nausea,vomiting,alopecia,headache	5	900085586
nna,neutropenia,nausea,vomiting,alopecia,loss of sleep,cough,constipation	4	800045063
nna,nausea	2	30105
nna,vomiting	2	62423
nna,neutropenia,nausea,vomiting,abdominal pain,guiddiness,suffocation,obstruction,diarrhoea,blackening at the base of the nail bed	9	900001234
nausea	1	900015091
nna,vomiting	2	78223
nna,nausea,hand and foot syndrome,alopecia,throbophlebitis	5	900011897
alopecia,anorexia,mouth ulcer,nausea	4	900046644
nna,nausea,anorexia,guiddiness,nail bed blackening of hand and sole,oral ulceration,sleep loss,alopecia	8	900063593
nna,anorexia,peripheral neuropathy	3	900053983
nna,bloating,wt.loss,anorexia,nausea,alopecia,headache	7	900085990
nna	1	900078207
nna,throbocytopenia,oral ulceration,nausea,vomiting,anorexia,abdpain,diarrohea,alopecia,headache,loss of sleep,blackening of nail bed,burning in eye	13	900010497
irritation in veins,nausea,vomiting,cough,diarroea	6	109706
nna,neutropenia,anorexia,alopecia,gastric upset,flatus formation	6	65180
nna,nausea,vomiting,alopecia	4	800017784
nna,abdpain,diarrhoea,thrombophlebitis,swelling of the lower limb joints,guiddiness,loss of sleep	6	900084408
nna	1	900098203
nna,nausea,vomiting,alopecia,headache,anorexia,blackening of foot and hands,pain in legs	7	900058963
vomiting	1	900012368
nna,thrombocytopenia,thrombophlebitis,alopecia	4	900013172
nna,alopecia,nausea,vomiting,neutropenia	5	900093094
nna,alopecia,neuropathy,neutropenia,nephrotoxicity,thrombophlebitis	6	900005448
nausea,vomiting,nna	3	900000626
nna,nausea,vomiting	3	900010476
vomiting,alopecia,nna,neutropenia,thrombocytopenia,gi bleeding,nephrotoxicity,hyponatremia	8	90003003
nausea,vomiting,alopecia,nna,anorexia,hepatotoxicity	6	65236
hairloss,nausea,vomiting,thrombophlebitis	4	900010045
nna,nausea,vomiting,burning in scalp and stomach,nephrotoxicity,alopecia,menses stopped for 4 months,thrombophlebitis,sleep disturbance,anorexia	10	900078891
nna,nausea,vomiting,alopecia,thrombophlebitis	5	900026936
nna,neutropenia	2	900093619
nna	1	108895
nna,hands and leg pain,peripheral neuropathy	3	900060683
nna,irritation to vein during infusion, nausea, vomiting, nephrotoxicity, tingling and numbness, pain in hands and legs, loss of sleep, diarrhoea.	10	900010400
nna,lymphopenia,severe wt. loss	3	900011974
alopecia,nna,nausea,vomiting,neutropenia	5	900004538
nna,irritation to vein during infusion, nausea, vomiting,oral mucositis,alopecia,oral mucositis,neutropenia	7	900057996
nna,nausea,vomiting,anorexia	4	900041861
nna,nausea,vomiting,alopecia,anorexia	5	900028010
nna,alopecia,anorexia,fever,neutropenia,hand and leg pain	6	8000144743
nna,hand foot syndrome	2	900062404
nna,nausea	2	9000676893
nna,rash(daunorubicin),neutropenia,nausea,vomiting,fever	6	900022544
nausea,vomiting,headache,abd pain,bloating,constipation,oral ulceration	7	900100978
nna,nausea,vomiting,injection site injury,anorexia	5	900073943
nna,nausea,vomiting	3	115775
loss of sleep	1	800019702

Symptoms	Count	ID
nna,neutropenia,nausea	3	800047260
nna,thrombocytopenia	2	900062100
nna,nausea,vomiting	3	9000111875
nausea,vomiting,loose motion,alopecia	4	90007100
nna,nausea,vomiting,fever,abdominal pain,headache,anal fissure,constipation,chills,sepsis	10	800035947
leukopenia,thrombocytopenia	2	900037707
nna,neutropenia,fever,abdominal pain,oral lesions	5	900003132
nausea,vomiting,nna	3	900132234
nna,nausea,vomiting,diarrhoea,hypermelanosis to chemo(either due to vcr or cyclophosphamide)	5	900012777
nna,guidiness,vomiting,hairloss,diarrhoea	5	900081503
nna,nausea,vomiting,diarrhoea(black stools),urine(black),hair loss,joint pain,lower limb pain	8	900016177
nna,hair loss	2	900046367
nna,nausea,vomiting,abdominal pain,oral leisions,alopecia,constipation,neutropenia,loss of sleep	9	900130777
nna,nausea,vomiting,neutropenia	4	900156611
nna,nausea,vomiting,abdominal pain	4	900108285
nna,nausea,vomiting,alopecia	4	900101670
nna,nausea,vomiting,neutropenia	3	900150245
nna,nausea,vomiting	10	900125206
nna,nausea,vomiting,thrombophlebitis,anorexia,sleepless,headache,tingling and numbness,wt loss,oligomenorrhoea	5	125037
nna,tingling and numbness,diarrhoea,sleeplessness,belching	6	900157395
nna,nausea,vomiting,pedaldema,irritation to veins,alopecia	5	800047451
nna,nausea,vomiting,anorexia,alopecia	6	900083714
nna,febrile neutropenia,sepsis,nephrotoxicity,loss of sleep	1	900143039
limb edema(thrombophlebitis)	4	900124335
nna,nausea,vomiting,alopecia	9	900010941
nna,nausea,vomiting,alopecia,oral leisions,abdominal pain,tingling,numbness,anorexia,diarrheoa	6	900129170
nna,hand foot syndrome,abdominal pain,diarrheoa,vomiting,headache	4	900110633
venous irritation,diarrhoea,tingling and numbness,alopecia	7	900117351
nna,pachy alopecia,nausea,vomiting,guidiness,thrombophlebitis,abdominal pain	2	800031416
fever,febrile neutropenia	9	900130493
nna,nausea,vomiting,thrombophlebitis,constipation,anorexia,alopecia,sleeploss,infection	5	900046598
thrombophlebitis,nna,nausea,vomiting,neutropenia	6	28750
nna,neutropenia,nausea,vomiting,diarrhoea,abdominalpain	5	9049945726
nna,alopecia,nausea,vomiting,neutropenia	4	2446546
nausea,vomiting,anorexia,diarrhea	6	976411734
nna,nausea,vomiting,diarrhoea,neutropenia,abdominalpain	7	9766343659
nna,nausea,vomiting,diarrhoea,neutropenia,abdominalpain,alopecia	5	9923382761
nna,nausea,vomiting,alopecia,nephrotoxicity,abdominalpain,alopecia	4	8007091958
nna,nausea,vomiting,alopecia,nephrotoxicity	6	288139
nna,nausea,vomiting,alopecia	4	902338162
nna,alopecia,neuropathy,neutropenia,thrombocytopenia,vomiting	4	900045321
nna,alopecia,nausea,vomiting	4	900043298
nna,alojpecia,nausea,vomiting	4	7658234
nna,nausea,vomiting,neutropenia	3	7673462
nausea,vomiting diarrhoea,anorexia	4	9850600325
vomiting,giddiness,diarrhoea	5	9850600346
nna,nausea,vomiting,interstitial pneumonitis	1	9785432165
nna,nausea,vomiting,interstitial pneumonitis,ascites	7	2325521
nna	7	7612384
nna,nausea,vomiting,alopecia,hand-foot syndrome,neutropenia	5	900084509
nna,nausea,vomiting,alopecia,thrombocytopenia,neutropenia,anorexia	6	09/54733
nna,nausea,vomiting,thrombophlebitis,neutropenia,alopecia		67441
nna,alopecia,neutropenia,anorexia,mucositis,thrombophlebitis		94609/09

Symptoms	Count	ID
nna,neutropenia,nausea,vomiting	4	900149982
nna,neutropenia,nausea,vomiting,alopecia	4	900014998
nausea,vomiting ,anorexia	3	900115619
nna,neutropenia,nausea,vomiting,peripheral neuropathy	6	812563
nna,neutropenia,nausea,vomiting,nephrotoxicity,anorexia	5	900115509
Neutropenia,Diarrhea ,nausea,vomiting,Alopecia ,peripheral neuropathy	8	81132456
nna,neutropenia,nausea,vomiting,bleeding	6	100005882
nausea,vomiting,abdominal Pain,constipation,nna	5	8000026957
nausea,vomiting ,alopecia	3	100013666
nna,nause,vomiting,diarrhea,apetite,anorexia,alopecia,scratching of hands and soles and boils,trombophlebitis	8	100002982
mucositis ,abdominal pain,	3	90011928
nausea,vomiting	2	100001492
nna,sepsis,neutropenia,nausea,vomiting	5	100002878
nna ,vomiting ,alopecia	3	90067548
nna,nausea,vomiting,brethlessness,pigmentation over neck,abdomen,thrombophlebitis,black stools,alopecia	9	90015210
nna,neutropenia	2	900012312
alopecia	1	900072530
nna	1	9001574
nna,peripheral neuropathy,extravasation of urine,neutropenia,constipation	5	90045390
vomiting	1	4134
nna	2	1000025076
nausea,vomiting	1	1000008625
nausea , vomiting , unconciousness,loss of sleep,convulsions,gtcs,hypotension ,death	6	1000546673
nausea,vomiting,neutropenia,anorexia	4	106058
nausea,vomiting,	2	900017981
nna,nausea,vomiting,neutropenia,mucositis,anorexia	6	900003425
nna,nausea,vomiting,neutropenia,mucositis,anorexia	6	900075343
nna,nausea,vomiting,neutropenia,mucositis,anorexia	6	9000140322
nna,peripheral neuropathy,anorexia,ascites,constipation	6	180213
nausea,peripheral neuropathy,weakness,anorexia,abdominal pain ,constipation, nephrotoxicity	7	900117559
nna,nausea,vomiting,neutropenia,mucositis,anorexia	7	900137491
nna,neutropenia,mucositis,diarrhea,nausea	5	900137491
nna,neutropenia,mucositis,diarrhea	4	900130778
anorexia,constipation,vomiting,alopecia,insomnia,peripheral neuropathy,mucositis,pleural effusion,alopecia	9	900130777
nna,nausea,vomiting	3	900006354
nausea,vomiting	2	900102439
nausea,vomiting,peripheral neuropathy,alopecia,insomnia,pleural effusion	6	100009320
alopecia,vomiting,peripheral neuropathy,alopecia,insomnia	5	900009036
nna,anorexia,hepatotoxicity	3	900112321
nna,ascites,diarrhoea,alopecia,anorexia,pleural effusion,vomiting	6	123684
nna,hypoproteinaemia,nausea,vomiting,anorexia	5	900120682
nna,neutropenia,alopecia,vomiting	4	90003452
fever,febrile neutropenia, chills,pealing of skin, pedal edema,alopecia,oral thrush	7	90004563
anorexia,constipation,vomiting,alopecia,insomnia,peripheral neuropathy,mucositis,pleural effusion,ascites	7	90035467

batch no.	date	associated drugs
	15/12/09	ideca or dexamethasone,iondem or ondensetron,irantac or ranitidine
	23/12/09	ideca,iondem,irantac
	16/12/09	irantac,ideca
	8/4/2010	ideca,iondem
	31/12/09	iondem,irantac
	16/01/10	iodem,irantac,
	15/03/10	iondem,irantac,ideca,ileucovorin
	17/12/09	iondem,irantac,ideca,ileucovorin
	9/9/2009	iondem,ideca,irantac,thrombophobe.ont.
	13/6/10	ionedm,ideca,irantac,tab.becosules or tablet B-complex
	1/7/2009	iondem,irantac,ideca,ileucovorin
	10/9/2009	iondem ,irantac, tab.bcosules,jleucovorin
	11/7/2009	iondem ,irantac, tab.bcosules,jleucovorin
	22/06/10	iondem,jleucovorin
	12/7/2009	iondem,ideca,imesna
	31/7/09	ionedem,ideca,irantac,tab.becosules,jleucovorin
	21/12/09	iondem,ideca,irantac
	12/12/2009	iondem,ideca,irantac
hk80586	14/02/10	iondem,irantac,iprednisolone,ideca,imetronidazole
	11/2/2010	iondem,ideca,jleucovorin
	21/02/10	iondem,ideca,irantac
	12/5/2010	iondem,irantac,ideca
	4/8/2009	iondem,irantac
jk80657	2/8/2009	iondem,irantac
	9/7/2009	iondem,irantac
	2/6/2010	idexamethasone,iondem
	20/7/09	itheophylline,ichlorpheniramine maleate,idexamethasone
	22/4/10	idexamethasone,itheophylline
	18/07/09	idexamethasone,iondem,irantac,tab.bplex or B-complex ,isodiumferrate
	14/04/10	ileucovorin,iondem,irantac
	20/7/09	ideca,irantac,iondem,iphenargan
	18/04/10	irantac,iondem
	13/04/10	irantac,iondem
	14/03/10	irantac,iondem
	20/5/10	multivitamin tablets,tramadol,i,aztreonam,jleucovorin
	9/9/2009	irantac,iondem
	20/10/09	iondem,irantac,ifilgrastim
	15/12/09	iondem ,ipantoprazole,imixtard,icefdroxil,jleucovorin
	31/05/10	icefdroxil,tab.valacyclovir,jondem
	23/07/10	tab.ciprofloxacin,iondem
	31/10/10	ileucovorin,iondem,jrantac
	21/10/10	irantac,iondem
	11/11/2010	iondem,tab.bplex,tab.multivitamin,jleucovorin
	11/8/2009	iondem,ichlorepheniramine maleate,ifilgrastim,imultivitamin
	9/12/2009	iondem,irantac
	10/7/2009	iondem,irantac,
	2/8/2009	iphenargan,iondem,ifilgrastim
	2/9/2009	iondem,tab.bplex,tab.multivitamin
	17/07/09	imannitol,iceftazidime,imeropenem,ivancomycin,iondem,ileucovorin
	2/7/2009	iondem,tab.rantac,jdeca,jleucovorin
	2/8/2009	irantac,iondem,jleucovorin
	15/1/10	iondem,ideca,jleucovorin

10/7/2009	tab.b.plex,imultivitamin,ileucovorin
Jul-09	tab.pyridoxine,iondem,tab.b plex,ileucovorin
7/8/2009	iondem,irantac
8/11/2009	iondem,irantac,ideca,ileucovorin
8/12/2009	iondem,irantac,tab.bcosules,ileucovorin
13/02/10	iondem,irantac
25/04/10	tab.b.plex,imultivitamin,ideca,irantac,iondem,ileucovorin
16/08/09	tab.bplex,imultivitamin,ileucovorin,iondem
16/08/09	tab.bplex,imultivitamin,tab.serratiopeptidase,iondem
17/07/09	irantac,iondem,ibplex,ifilgrastim
17/12/09	idilantin,ibplex,tab.amoxycillin,tab.ondem
17/06/10	iondem,irantac
30/08/09	iondem,irantac
30/09/09	iondem,irantac
27/10/09	iondem,irantac,ileucovorin
30/11/09	iondem,irantac
8/9/2009	tabpantoprazole,iondem,irantac
29/05/10	iondem,ideca
30/08/09	iondem,ideca,oracib gel,i leucovorin
25/09/09	imannitol,irantac,ideca,iphenergan,ont.thrombophobe
25/08/09	irantac,iondem,tab.bplex,ifilgrastim
9/11/2009	irantac,iondem,tab.bplex
17/07/09	ivancomycin,ont.betadine ,tab.bplex,iceftazidime,irantac,ileucovorin
8/10/2009	iondem,irantac
8/7/2009	ibplex,imultivitamin,iserratiopeptidase,iondem,ileucovorin
8/10/2009	ibplex,iondem,irantac,ideca,ileucovorin
11/7/2009	icollistin,ideca,ileucovorin
11/12/2009	iondem,tab.granisetron,imultivitamin,ileucovorin
12/9/2009	iondem,irantac,ideca,iphenargan,tab.amlodipine,ileucovorin
2/8/2009	iondem,irantac
2/9/2009	iondem,irantac
15/08/09	iphenargan,iondem,itramadol,tab.bplex,ifilgrastim
7/9/2009	irantac,iondem,tab.bplex
8/8/2009	irantac,iondem,tab.bplex
28/8/9	irantac,iondem,tab.bplex
14/07/09	ideca,irantac,iondem,iphenargan
14/8/9	irantac,iondem,tab.bplex,ifilgrastim
14/08/09	imultivitamin,tab.bplex,iondem,irantac
10/8/2009	irantac,iondem,ibplex
14/10/09	irantac,iondem,ibplex
2/8/2009	irantac,iondem,ibplex
2/7/2009	irantac,iondem,ibplex
8/7/2009	irantac,iondem,ibplex
21/12/09	irantac,iondem,ibplex
25/12/09	irantac,iondem,tab.bplex
20/08/09	irantac,iondem,tab.bplex
23/5/09	irantac,iondem,tab.bplex
14/08/09	irantac,iondem,ibplex
13/2/10	irantac,tab.ondem,tab diclofenacsodium
10/9/2009	irantac,iondem,ibplex
2/8/2009	irantac,iondem,tab bplex
12/11/2009	irantac,iondem,ibplex
10/9/2009	iondem,ideca,ipantoprazole,ibplex

12/9/2009	irantac,iondem,ibplex
14/09/09	irantac,iondem,tab.bplex
13/10/09	irantac,iondem,tab.bplex
23/09/09	irantac,iondem,tab.bplex
29/7/08	iomeprazole,ibplex,iondem,ileucovorin ,ifilgrastim
16/11/09	tabciplox,ileucovorin,imultivitamin,ifilgrastim
26/08/09	iondem,ideca,irantac
26/10/09	iondem,irantac
28/11/09	icefotaxim,irantac,iondem,imetronidazole,tabfolic acid,ifilgrastim
20/08/09	iondem,irantac
31/10/09	iondem,irantac
14/11/09	iondem,irantac
12/11/2009	irantac,iondem,ideca,phenargan
6/4/2010	iondem,irantac
20/12/09	iondem,irantac
26/10/09	iondem,irantac
11/12/2009	iondem,irantac
19/10/09	iondem,irantac,ideca
22/11/09	iondem,irantac,tab.bcosules,ileucovorin,ifilgrastim
2/5/2010	iondem,irantac
23/07/08	iondem,irantac
22/08/09	iondem,irantac
21/09/09	iondem,irantac,tab.bcosules,ifilgrastim,icefoperazone
22/11/09	iondem,ifurosemide
6/11/2009	iondem,tab.rantac
6/11/2009	iondem,irantac,tab.becosules
8/10/2009	tab.becosules,ileucovorin,ifilgrastim
15/10/09	ideca,irantac,iondem,iphenargan,tab.becosules
26/10/09	iondem,irantac,ont.thrombophobe
12/9/2009	iondem,irantac
18/12/08	iondem,irantac,ideca,ifilgrastim
10/10/2009	iondem,irantac,ipantoprazole
11/11/2009	iondem,irantac,ifilgrastim
13/1/10	iondem,irantac,ifilgrastim,ipantoprazole
15/12/09	iondem,irantac
3/2/2010	iondem,ideca,ifilgrastim
27/1/10	iondem,ideca
30/9/09	iondem,ideca
13/11/09	iondem,ideca
15/04/10	iondem,ideca
18/10/09	iondem,ideca,ifilgrastim
16/09/09	iondem,ideca
12/9/2009	iondem,ideca
27/04/10	iondem,ideca
18/05/10	iondem,ideca
21/05/10	iondem,ideca
3/2/2010	iondem,ideca
1/12/2009	iondem,ideca
23/08/09	i odem,i deca,irantac
15/08/09	iondem,ideca
3/7/2009	iondem,ideca,irantac
24/07/09	iondem,irantac,ideca
5/8/2009	iondem,irantac,ideca

12/7/2009	iondem,irantac,ideca
15/3/10	igranisetron,ideca,irantac
8/4/2010	iondem,irantac,ideca
12/1/2010	iondem,ideca
8/10/2009	iondem,ideca
20/1/10	iondem,ideca
12/1/2010	iondem,ideca
13/7/09	iondem,ideca
15/9/09	iondem,irantac
25/12/09	iondem ,ideca,irantac,iavil
8/4/2010	iondem,ideca,irantac
12/2/2010	iondem,irntac,t dilantin
8/4/2010	iondem,irantac,iprednisolone,ideca,iceftriaxone,imetronidazole
20/06/10	ideca,iondem,irantac,l,phenargan
17/2/10	icisplatin,ietoposide,ibleomycin
18/2/10	icisplatin,i5fu
2/2/2010	icisplatin
20/2/10	iondem
23/9/09	iondem,irantac,ileucovorin
20/12/09	iondem,irantac
4/6/2010	tab,ondem
4/6/2010	iondem
5/1/2010	iondem,irantac.ideca.isod.valproate,isomatostatin,igm-csf
20/11/2009	iodem,irantac,
13/1/2010	iondem,irantac
10/1/2010	iondem,rantac,ideca,ileucovorin
21/6/2010	iondem,irantac,ideca
21/6/2010	iondem,irantac,ideca
15/2/2010	iondem,irantac,ideca
20/1/2010	iondem,iphenargan,irantac
12/1/2010	iondem,irantac,ideca
20/1/2010	iondem,irantac,ideca
20/2/2010	iondem,irantac,ideca
20/2/2010	iondem,irantac,ideca,ileucovorin,isaphgul
15/7/09	iondem,irantac,ideca
22/3/2010	iondem,irantac,ideca
12/12/2009	iondem,irantac,tab.bplex,t vitamin
10/2/2010	igranisetron,ideca,irantac
14/10/09	ideca,iondem,irantac,l,phenargan
13/10/09	ideca,iondem,irantac,l,phenargan
30/10/09	ideca,iondem,irantac,l,phenargan
9/1/2010	ideca,iondem,irantac,l,phenargan
21/01/2010	ideca,iondem,irantac,l,phenargan,ipiperacillin,itazobactum,t.vibact,trivotril
20/01/2010	ideca,iondem,irantac,ifurosemide,iceftriaxone

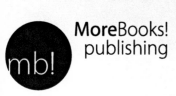
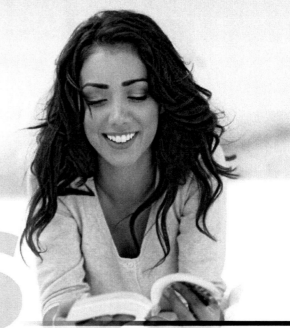

Lightning Source UK Ltd.
Milton Keynes UK
UKOW03f2347210314

228639UK00001B/67/P